The Situational Judgement Test

DATE DUE

PRINTED IN U.S.A.

Get ahead!

The Situational Judgement Test

Nishanthan Mahesan MBBS BSc (Hons)
Foundation Trainee, North East Thames
Foundation School, UK

Sirazum M. Choudhury MBBS BSc (Hons)
Foundation Trainee, North Central Thames
Foundation School, UK

Janice Rymer MD FRCOG FRANZCOG FHEA
Dean of Undergraduate Medicine and Professor
of Gynaecology, King's College London

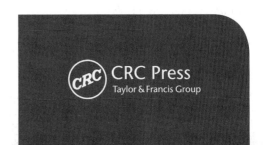
CRC Press
Taylor & Francis Group

CRC Press
Taylor & Francis Group
6000 Broken Sound Parkway NW, Suite 300
Boca Raton, FL 33487-2742

No claim to original U.S. Government works
Printed and bound by CPI Group (UK) Ltd, Croydon, CR0 4YY
International Standard Book Number: 978-1-4441-7660-5 (Softcover)

Library of Congress Cataloging-in-Publication Data

Catalog record is available from the Library of Congress

Visit the Taylor & Francis Web site at
http://www.taylorandfrancis.com

and the CRC Press Web site at
http://www.crcpress.com

Foreword

Medical education has undergone enormous changes over the last two decades. Gone are the days of didactic lectures. Teaching is now more student-centred with an emphasis on students taking on the responsibility of advancing their own education with self-directed and problem-based learning. The teaching methodologies have changed, not only to give the students a more intellectually stimulating experience but also to reflect the changing practice of medicine. Patients are now more involved in decisions about their own treatment and are more questioning about their medication, often asking for the evidence base on which these decisions are made. On top of this, with faster travel across the world, the actual practice of medicine has changed with diseases becoming more global and, with the inevitable movement of people across countries, a richer mixture of different cultures within societies. Thus new doctors have the challenging task of not only having the appropriate medical knowledge but will also have to meet difficult scenarios which will test their professional and personal attributes, attitudes and preconceptions. A very challenging task!

The General Medical Council (GMC) and medical schools work towards producing curricula that are more focussed and appropriate for the populations we serve. It is therefore inevitable that as the curricula change, the actual methodology for assessment of students needs to be addressed to reflect these innovations.

One such assessment tool is the Situational Judgement Test (SJT), which has been designed to examine the awareness and response of trainees to these difficult scenarios. It is more objective in assessing the desired attributes of a safe and competent doctor, removing the bias involved in previous forms of assessment.

This book is intended for medical students and foundation trainees. It is designed as a revision book to help the trainee through a set of intellectual mental processes in order to reach a correct answer. In difficult situations there are often no correct answers but those that involve a balance of ethics, judgement and professionalism. It is all about assessing and balancing a situation to reach the most suitable answer to the dilemma posed. The book is based on the views of experienced clinicians. It contains plenty of questions covering a wide array of professional dilemmas. I found these most testing but also fun to do!

The book also contains several dedicated chapters containing tips for trainees to assist them in answering the SJT questions. It gives some background information on GMC guidance and references on difficult ethical issues encountered in the daily duty of a doctor such as consent, capacity and confidentiality.

This book will be very useful for the trainee and the more senior medical student. The SJT will be taken by all final year medical students and the results will count towards the allocation of foundation posts. It will also be a refresher aid for doctors at any stage of their career. It is written by foundation trainees who have experienced the examination as well as experienced clinicians. I am sure it will be an excellent new addition to books that help us to revise for different examinations.

Professor Parveen J Kumar CBE BSc MD FRCP FRCPE
Professor of Medicine and Education, Bart's and the London School
of Medicine and Dentistry, Queen Mary, University of London
President of the Royal Society of Medicine
Co-author of Kumar and Clark's *Clinical Medicine*

Preface

Medical students will only have had limited exposure to the Situational Judgement Test (SJT) until this crucial juncture in their medical careers. The results of this examination carry a great deal of significance and contribute towards what ultimately determines where they will work as doctors.

Rather than being a test of clinical knowledge or technical skills, this test aims to elicit the essential attributes of a successful foundation trainee by presenting challenging and realistic scenarios that assess various professional competencies. Proponents of this examination highlight that such a test cannot be revised for; indeed, clinical experience is key to developing the skills and attitudes required to answer these questions. This book is intended as a preparatory tool for the SJT and offers an organised and focused study of the aspects of clinical practice that are to be assessed. The initial chapters are a compilation of basic ethical concepts and GMC guidance on the most commonly encountered scenarios, and a log of prerequisite knowledge that will assist with answering these types of questions.

This book offers a logical approach to questions and details the sequence to deriving the correct order of answers. Each answer is then backed with justification drawn from official guidance.

The questions and answers included in this book are examples and based on the expected style and content of the SJT examination. The model answers and justifications are based on the authors' interpretation of current information and guidance on the relevant issues. As such, the answers found in this book may deviate from the model answers in the examination for similar scenarios.

We hope that this book offers you the preparation you require to succeed in this examination.

On behalf of everyone involved in the production of this book, we would like to take this opportunity to wish you the best of luck for this examination and your future medical career.

Nishanthan Mahesan, Sirazum M. Choudhury and Janice Rymer

Contents

1: Introduction

THE SITUATIONAL JUDGEMENT TEST

The practice of medicine is both rewarding and intellectually stimulating. Doctors are placed in a unique position of enormous privilege, with patients sharing their most intimate details, allowing the clinician to fully explore the presenting complaint and address all aspects of their care.

Seeing a myriad of patients from all walks of life and a variety of cultures, while treating each as an individual and acknowledging what is important to them, continues to excite and challenge us. The daily activities of a doctor are therefore highly variable, with novel cases presenting to even the most experienced clinicians. Often challenging scenarios arise and guidance is needed on the most appropriate way to approach them while upholding the principles of the profession.

The Situational Judgement Test (SJT) is designed to highlight these personal and professional dilemmas, and examine the response of foundation trainees to these scenarios. The questions aim to portray common situations that arise and test the essential attributes of a foundation doctor. While the available responses to a given question may not always be ideal, exploring the manner in which an individual prioritises and assesses the suitability of particular actions can help paint a picture of the level of understanding and intuition that the prospective doctor has. The most challenging aspect of this assessment is demonstrating the flexibility required to take the ethical considerations and guidance offered by the General Medical Council (GMC), consider them, and then apply them to a given scenario.

Since it has a more linear and objective basis of examination, the SJT removes the bias associated with marking the forms of assessment that had previously been used in this application process. While it is difficult to prepare for such an examination, an awareness of a doctor's priorities in frequently encountered scenarios will aid in identifying the common underlying themes and the accepted manner in which to deal with them. Appreciating the nine domains of the successful foundation trainee, which are visited in the next chapter, will further help to direct the doctor's attention to the more pressing actions in a scenario.

The SJT has recently been introduced to Foundation Training, underscoring its increasing popularity in the medical profession as a tool to assess the desired attributes of a safe and competent doctor. The questions in this book are broadly based on the authors' own experiences as doctors.

Others are extrapolated from important situations arising in the clinical setting. The guidance on these issues is based on the experience of senior colleagues with a specialist interest in the relevant field, in addition to the guidance produced by the GMC and other professional bodies.

The model answers in this book are based on the views and experiences of clinicians and providers of medical education, similar to those in the formal examination. This book is intended as a learning tool to develop the right thought processes in reaching the correct set of answers. As such, memorising answers in each scenario is inadvisable as you are unlikely to encounter precisely the same scenario and set of options in the actual examination. Instead, understanding the justification for the correct ranking of the possible responses, in light of the scenario and the other options available, is likely to provide the best preparation for the SJT.

THE EDUCATIONAL PERFORMANCE MEASURE

In addition to the examination component of the application process, the Educational Performance Measure (EPM) is used to allocate points that are combined with the SJT score to produce an overall score that is used to rank each candidate. The scoring for the EPM consists of three separate parts:

1. **Medical school performance**, which provides a decile score. Applicants at a given medical school are ranked against one another and given a score depending on which group they fall into. The top 10 per cent will be awarded the maximum mark for this section, and the points awarded will decrease in increments with each subsequent 10-per-cent group. Deciles are allocated using local policy, which is determined by the medical school that a candidate belongs to. Further information on this may be sought from your medical school.
2. **Additional degrees**: This includes Bachelor's, Master's and Doctorate degrees. Points are awarded for the classification of a degree, with more points offered for a first-class honours degree than for a third-class degree.
3. **Publications, presentations and prizes.**
   a. **Publications**: In order to gain points for publications, they must be peer-reviewed and have a PubMed ID (PMID). Alternatively, a letter of evidence to state that the work has been accepted for publication and is 'in press' for an article that has a PMID is also acceptable.
   b. **Presentations**: In order to gain points for presentations, they must be oral or poster presentations given at a national or international conference, and hosted by a recognised professional medical body.
   c. **Prizes**: In order to gain points for prizes, they must be national or international educational prizes which are awarded by an organisation that is not student-led. Points are not awarded for bursaries, scholarships, research grants, university prizes or elective awards. The prize awarded must be the first prize.

The precise scoring system for the EPM is likely to change each year and additional conditions for each component may also apply. The current criteria may be found from the latest 'Foundation Applicant's Handbook'. This, in addition to further information on the entire application process, may be found on the Foundation Programme website.

THE FOUNDATION PROGRAMME APPLICATION SYSTEM

As part of the Foundation Programme Application System (FPAS), candidates are required to rank Foundation Schools in order of preference. While the algorithm changes each year, the principle of allocating a candidate to their preferred Foundation School remains the same.

Once analysed, the SJT and EPM marks are combined to provide an overall score for each candidate. This score is ranked against every other applicant involved in the process. The highest scoring candidates are allocated to their most preferred choices. Once a particular Foundation School's vacancies have been filled, the algorithm is used to best-match remaining candidates to their next highest ranking Foundation School.

Once allocated to a particular Foundation School, candidates are required to undergo a local application process that is responsible for assigning specific hospitals and rotations. This can once again be influenced by a candidate's mark from the combined SJT and EPM score, but may also involve additional interviews or other assessments.

This entire application process usually occurs during the final year of medical studies.

2: Analysis of SJT Questions

The Situational Judgement Test (SJT) will comprise around 70 questions to be taken in 2 hours 20 minutes. This allows for 2 minutes to be spent on each question. Organisation and effective time management are therefore vital during the examination.

Of the total number of questions, 60 will count towards the final score, while the remaining 10 are pilot questions which may be used in future years. The 10 pilot questions will be indistinguishable from the assessed questions and are distributed throughout the paper.

The two possible question formats in the exam are:

1. **Ranking questions**: Rank five possible responses in the most appropriate order. This type of question will account for two-thirds of the paper.
2. **Multiple response questions**: Select the three most appropriate responses for the situation. This type of question will account for one-third of the paper.

When presented with the same scenario, answers may differ slightly, so partial deviations from the model answer may still be given credit. In principle, the further someone deviates from the model answer, the less credit their answer is given. The specific scoring system for each question type is outlined below.

In general, the responses given for each question can be broadly arranged as appropriate or inappropriate. You may be able to formulate two groups; those that are appropriate, and those that are inappropriate. The ranking questions inevitably take longer to consider given that comparisons have to be made between each response, particularly within each of the two groups that you have just created. In contrast, when considering the multiple response questions, the inappropriate responses can simply be excluded. You will be left to choose three responses out of the four or five remaining, and comparisons between individual options need not be made with the multiple response questions.

Particular attention should be paid to the underlying theme of each question. Identifying the theme, or themes where more than one is examined, is key to approaching the responses in the correct fashion. Questions should always be screened for any threats to patient welfare, as these are of overriding consequence. Other themes may also be present and these must be ranked against one another, and the available options chosen accordingly. For instance, discussing a patient on the way to the car at the end of a busy shift may ensure that you are able to exit swiftly and preserve a good work/life balance while providing an adequate handover, but you must identify that this may threaten a patient's confidentiality if the conversation is overheard. Therefore, maintaining patient confidentiality overrides the preservation of a satisfactory work/life balance.

Of equal importance is the need for the responses to be carefully read and assessed. Just as with any multiple choice question, small details in the available options must be noticed and considered carefully. Minute variations can change a response that initially appears appropriate into one that is unsuitable upon closer inspection.

With practice you will appreciate that while the scenarios change, many of the underlying themes are the same, and thus your priorities in these situations will remain unchanged.

RANKING QUESTIONS

Ranking the available options

In these questions you will be given a scenario and asked to rank typically five options from the most appropriate action to the least appropriate action. Here is an example:

You are a foundation year 1 (FY1) doctor on a medical on-call. You arrive at a cardiac arrest, where you find an anaesthetist managing the airway and two nurses performing chest compressions. The anaesthetist requests that you intubate the patient, while she prepares the ventilator. You have only intubated a patient once in the past and are concerned about doing this without direct supervision.

Rank in order the following actions in response to this situation (1 = Most appropriate; 5 = Least appropriate).

A Tell one of the nurses to contact the medical registrar on-call.
B Refuse to intubate the patient.
C Find the medical registrar on-call yourself.
D Ask the anaesthetist to instruct you on setting up the ventilator, while she intubates the patient.
E Ask the anaesthetist to instruct you on intubating the patient, while she sets up the ventilator.

This question is one of the worked examples in the next chapter where more information on how to deal with this type of scenario can be found.

As mentioned above, when considering this type of question, you should read the question and responses with the aim of identifying the themes that are being assessed. When reviewing the available responses, there may be those that are clearly the most or least appropriate. These options should be assigned their rank accordingly and eliminated from further consideration. The remaining options can then be ranked against one another and placed in the appropriate position. With practice, common red flags will be picked up more readily which would demote a particular response.

Scoring for ranking questions

A total of 20 marks is available for each ranking question. For each of the five responses that you put down, a maximum of four marks is available. Partial marks will be awarded for near misses; the mark you are awarded for a response decreases as it deviates further from the model answer. There is no negative marking, though attributing the same rank to more than one response will result in a mark of 0 for each response that is tied.

MULTIPLE RESPONSE QUESTIONS

Selecting the most appropriate responses

The second type of question requires you to select the most appropriate response in a given scenario. You will be asked to choose typically the three most appropriate responses. There is no need to rank the options you have chosen. Here is an example:

> You are approaching the end of a long shift. You have arranged to meet some friends but you are already running late. Your colleague, who is supposed to be taking over, still has not arrived on the ward for you to hand over.
>
> Choose the THREE most appropriate actions to take in this situation.

A Check with medical staffing to ensure your colleague has not called in sick.

B Hand over to the registrar who has just started his shift if he is willing to accept the responsibility.

C Instruct the nurses to tell your colleague to call you when he arrives for the handover and leave the ward.

D Tell your consultant that your colleague was late and it resulted in you staying unnecessarily.

E Call your colleague to determine why he is delayed.

F Cover the shift until your colleague arrives and offer to stay for the entire shift if your colleague is indeed unwell.

G Leave when your shift ends as you have made a commitment to your friends.

H Leave a detailed handover sheet on the ward.

This question can also be found as one of the worked examples in the next chapter, where more information on how to deal with this type of scenario can be found.

The most appropriate response may be immediately obvious, but you will need to use your experience and reasoning to rule out other options and determine those which are most suitable. It is also worth noting that none of the available options may be what you would ideally do in a given scenario and therefore you will then need to choose the best available options from those provided. Once you have chosen the three most appropriate options, you should ensure that they are indeed the most suitable, and that they do not contradict one another.

Scoring for multiple response questions

A total of 12 marks is available for each multiple response question. You are required to pick the three most appropriate actions, and each correct answer attracts four marks. No partial marks are available for this question type. Once again, there is no negative marking, but choosing more than the stated number of responses will attract a score of 0 marks for the entire question.

THE NINE DOMAINS OF A SUCCESSFUL FOUNDATION DOCTOR

The questions that you will encounter in the exam aim to test the attributes which are required in a successful foundation trainee. A job analysis that was conducted on the role of an FY1 identified nine essential professional attributes, and the questions in the exam will be drawn from these.

The nine domains which were identified are as follows:

1. **Commitment to professionalism**: Appreciating the importance of upholding the reputation of the profession by acting with integrity in interactions with patients and other professionals. Being willing to address matters surrounding the professionalism of others and issues that threaten patient safety. Understanding that the reputation of the profession is the foundation upon which the doctor–patient partnership is built.

2. **Coping with pressure**: Possessing the ability to manage pressure. In addition to effective time management, ensuring emotional and physical well-being in light of the stresses of the profession. Developing suitable preventative strategies in aid of addressing identified issues in the long term.

3. **Effective communication**: Adapting communication style to suit the needs of the audience, combining verbal and non-verbal approaches where appropriate. Conveying information accurately and concisely among other members of the healthcare team, as well as patients and their relatives.

4. **Learning and professional development**: Ensuring knowledge and skills are up to date. Actively seeking and engaging in learning opportunities to develop and further these competencies. Being open and accepting of feedback that is received on performance, and willing to learn from others. Participation in the teaching of others.

5. **Organisation and planning**: Organising the resources that are available to you in an effective manner, and delegating where necessary. Anticipating and prioritising problems and pre-empting them where possible. Effectively managing time to maximise productivity. Keeping accurate and legible records.

6. **Patient focus**: Recognising the importance of the patient as the central focus of care. Affording patients an empathetic relationship, promoting trust and facilitating a partnership between doctor and patient. Paying consideration to families and relatives, and ensuring that the confidentiality of the patient is continually safe-guarded.

7. **Problem solving and decision making**: Demonstrating initiative and flexibility in dealing with challenges. Recognising obstacles to patient care and negotiating them to provide optimal management. Appreciating the importance of making necessary decisions and knowing when to defer such decisions to senior colleagues.

8. **Self-awareness and insight**: Understanding the limits of one's own abilities and avoidance of working beyond clinical competencies. Demonstrating insight into occasions where matters need to be escalated and senior help sought. Recognising the ethical implications of actions and being able to justify such decisions.

9. **Working effectively as part of a team**: Recognising that all members of a team have an important contribution to make to patient care. Understanding the role of others and promoting the creation of an open and encouraging atmosphere ensures that all members are fully supported.

You will notice that many of these overlap with the 'Person Specification', which is available on the Foundation Programme website and the 'Duties of a Doctor', outlined by the General Medical Council (GMC). An awareness of these will assist in identifying the specific attributes which are examined by a given SJT question.

3: Common Topics in SJT Questions

The questions in the exam will be based around scenarios which you are likely to face as a foundation year 1 (FY1) doctor. They aim to assess your professional attributes by examining how you would respond in some of the challenging situations you may encounter, and will require you to draw on the experiences you have acquired through medical school.

The following are examples of the kinds of questions you are likely to face. A suggested approach for answering is given beneath each question, with reference to the guidance provided by the General Medical Council (GMC) on what is expected of doctors in these situations.

EXAMPLE 1

You are an FY1 on a medical on-call. You arrive at a cardiac arrest, where you find an anaesthetist managing the airway and two nurses performing chest compressions. The anaesthetist requests that you intubate the patient, while she prepares the ventilator. You have only intubated a patient once in the past and are concerned about doing this without direct supervision.

Rank in order the following actions in response to this situation (1 = Most appropriate; 5 = Least appropriate).

A Tell one of the nurses to contact the medical registrar on-call.
B Refuse to intubate the patient.
C Find the medical registrar on-call yourself.
D Ask the anaesthetist to instruct you on setting up the ventilator, while she intubates the patient.
E Ask the anaesthetist to instruct you on intubating the patient, while she sets up the ventilator.

Approach to question
When presented with a scenario, it is important to determine whether there is potential risk to patient safety. Such scenarios may include the actions or inaction of colleagues, or the state a patient is in when you are called to a ward. If the welfare of the patient is compromised, your immediate response should address this first. Therefore it is important to evaluate every question for any potential harm to the patient. If the welfare of the patient is compromised, the first priority should be to attend to this, while subsequent actions can be to prevent similar events in the future.

It is also important to have an awareness of your own limitations and know when to ask for help. This includes not performing procedures that are outside your competencies. When answering this question you must balance treating the patient for their condition, with performing a procedure that may cause harm.

This appears to be a daunting question at first glance. However, approaching each option in turn with an awareness of your priorities helps to decipher the correct ranking order for the responses. In this scenario, performing the procedure incorrectly may result in further harm to the patient, exacerbating the situation. Thus the best options involve refraining from intubating the patient yourself, while ensuring the patient is treated. Considering this, it is most appropriate to ask the anaesthetist to intubate while you offer to help with other tasks (Option D). You should not perform the procedure yourself, as you have not reached the required competency and may cause further harm. Asking one of the nurses who is not performing chest compressions to contact the medical registrar (Option A) will ensure that a doctor with significant experience arrives on the scene with the short-term loss of a nurse. This is better than seeking out the registrar yourself (Option C), whereby the resuscitating team will be short of one skilled person for an indefinite period of time, which may prove detrimental to the patient.

After considering these options, you are left with refusing to intubate the patient (Option B) and intubating the patient yourself under verbal instruction (Option E). Given that it is more important not to cause harm than to summon the registrar, refusing to intubate is more appropriate. It is, however, not as suitable an answer as Option D, which ensures that the patient is treated. The remaining response (Option E) is clearly the most inappropriate, being the only option in which you conduct the intubation, and this poses a risk of causing the patient significant harm. Thus this is the worst answer and should be ranked last.

Example 1 answer is: D, B, A, C, E.

Guidance on Example 1: Patient welfare

This scenario highlights the need to ensure patient safety at all times. The GMC's 'Good Medical Practice' publication, states that 'Good doctors make the care of their patients their first concern' and that 'in providing care you must recognise and work within the limits of your competence'.

You must therefore take adequate action if patient safety is affected, or if there is potential for this to occur. If a situation arises which is beyond your clinical competencies, you must call for senior help.

In instances where errors are made, it is imperative to first reverse or limit the harm experienced by the patient, where possible. Once the issue of patient harm has been addressed, it is important to be upfront with the patient about any errors, even if they were unintentional, and irrespective of the degree of harm caused to the patient. The GMC states that 'You must act immediately to put matters right', and, following on from this:

You should offer an apology and explain fully and promptly to the patient what has happened, and the likely short-term and long-term effects.

EXAMPLE 2

One of your close FY1 colleagues confides in you that they have been finding work quite challenging and have grown increasingly dependent on alcohol. He asks you not to tell anyone.

Rank in order the following actions in response to this situation (1 = Most appropriate; 5 = Least appropriate).

A Agree with your colleague and not tell anyone.
B Reassure your colleague and suggest that he speaks to his registrar.
C Tell the nurses on the ward what has been happening.
D Report your colleague to the GMC as you believe patients are being put at risk.
E Tell your colleague's registrar without informing him.

Approach to question

It is important to maintain good working relationships with your colleagues. However, as mentioned in the previous example, the welfare of the patient needs to take priority. When reading the question, you must determine whether there is potential for patient care to be compromised.

In this scenario, this may be the case and so appropriate action is required. Therefore, doing nothing (Option A) is not a suitable response. When the work ethic of colleagues is inadequate or inappropriate, it is advisable to deal with problems locally before escalating these issues with the relevant bodies. It is therefore appropriate to discuss these issues with your colleague and encourage him to seek help (Option B), before informing your seniors directly (Option E).

Telling the nurses on the ward (Option C) does not deal with the issue and may adversely affect your relationship with your colleague, and is therefore the least appropriate response. Reporting your colleague to the GMC (Option D) and agreeing with your colleague to conceal his dependence (Option A) are both inadvisable. However, you must act if you believe patient safety is being put at risk, so Option D is preferable to not doing anything (Option A).

Example 2 answer is: B, E, D, A, C.

Guidance on Example 2: Working with colleagues

Maintaining good working relationships with colleagues is important. Patient safety must, however, supersede this. If problems do arise, aim to deal with matters locally before involving senior parties. The GMC's 'Good Medical Practice' paragraph 43 states:

You must protect patients from risk of harm posed by another colleague's conduct, performance or health. The safety of patients must come first at all times. If you have concerns that a colleague may not be fit to practise, you must take appropriate steps without delay, so that the concerns are investigated and patients protected when necessary.

The situation is therefore best handled by approaching it sensitively to attempt to preserve your working relationship with your colleague, while taking necessary measures to protect patients. However, when this is not possible you must be clear that protecting patients comes first, even at the cost of compromising your relationship with a colleague.

EXAMPLE 3

A taxi driver under your care is diagnosed with epilepsy and has been informed that he should stop driving due to his medical condition. On discharge, you explain the reasons for this and advise that he should inform the DVLA himself. On your way to work the following week, you notice him in his car picking up passengers.

Choose the THREE most appropriate actions to take in this situation.

A Chase after him to warn his passengers.
B Get into the car with him and confront him regarding his driving.
C Call his wife to warn her that her partner should immediately cease driving.
D Call the police as he poses a risk to other road users.
E Inform the DVLA.
F Call the patient and remind him of your advice and his obligations.
G Book another appointment to see him urgently.
H Tell your consultant about what you have seen.

Approach to question

This scenario concerns patient confidentiality and disclosure of sensitive information. Such disclosure is likely to adversely affect the doctor–patient relationship and impact upon the trust that has been built. However, one must consider and weigh this against the potential harm to others, in this instance fellow road users.

In this scenario, the patient has been diagnosed with epilepsy. If he was to have another seizure at the wheel of his taxi, this would place his passengers and other road users at risk of harm. Therefore, the most appropriate action would be to inform him to cease driving immediately (Option B). Such action would maintain confidentiality, preserve trust and remove the risk to the public.

The doctor should call the patient and make every reasonable effort to persuade him to stop driving (Option F). Booking an urgent appointment (Option G) could also be considered, but would not directly address the situation and would delay cessation of the patient's driving. Calling the patient's wife (Option C) is not ideal but minimises the breach of confidentiality and promptly limits the harm to the patient and public.

Warning the patient's passengers (Option A) would constitute a breach of confidentiality and is not suitable. Calling the DVLA (Option E) is not appropriate at this stage as the patient should be offered every reasonable effort to persuade him to stop driving. Informing the police (Option D) also constitutes a breach of confidentiality that would be excessive in light of other options. Informing the consultant (Option H) is advisable and preserves confidentiality, however, this would not resolve the situation.

Example 3 answer is: B, C, F.

Guidance on Example 3: Confidentiality

This question highlights the importance of patient confidentiality and covers the dilemma of having to weigh the patient's right to confidentiality against the public interest. Confidentiality issues are broad-ranging; knowledge of how confidentiality relates to adults and young people, issues surrounding capacity, driving rules, and when to break confidentiality, is important. Each of these will now be explored.

Confidentiality issues in adults

You must always aim to maintain patient confidentiality wherever possible. The GMC publication 'Confidentiality' states:

> *Confidentiality is central to trust between doctors and patients. Without assurances about confidentiality, patients may be reluctant to seek medical attention or to give doctors the information they need in order to provide good care.*

There are instances where this issue is complicated by the presence of family members who wish to discuss or share information with you regarding a patient that is under your care. The same publication by the GMC states:

> *You should establish with the patient what information they want you to share, who with, and in what circumstances.*

In addition:

> *If anyone close to the patient wants to discuss their concerns about the patient's health, you should make it clear to them that, while it is not a breach of confidentiality to listen to their concerns, you cannot guarantee that you will not tell the patient about the conversation.*

However:

> *You should not refuse to listen to a patient's partner, carers or others on the basis of confidentiality. Their views or the information they provide might be helpful in your care of the patient.*

This is therefore a complex area that requires you to determine the patient's wishes regarding who you can discuss sensitive information with, while taking note of information that is provided to you that might be helpful in their care.

Confidentiality issues in those that lack capacity

A patient must be assumed to have capacity, unless it is established that they lack capacity. Assessment of a patient's capacity must be performed at the time a particular decision needs to be made. In addition, if a patient lacks capacity to make a decision on a particular occasion, they cannot be assumed to lack capacity to make any decisions at all.

The Mental Capacity Act 2005 states that a person lacks capacity if they are unable to make a decision for themselves in relation to a matter, due to an impairment or disturbance in the functioning of the mind or brain. It states that a person is unable to make a decision for themselves if they are unable to do at least one of the following:

1. Understand the information relevant to the decision
2. Retain that information
3. Use or weigh that information as part of making the decision
4. Communicate that decision (through any means).

It is worth noting that a patient cannot be considered unable to make a decision because they have made an unwise choice regarding their treatment.

If a patient does lack capacity, the GMC publication 'Confidentiality' states:

> Unless they indicate otherwise, it is reasonable to assume that patients would want those closest to them to be kept informed of their general condition and prognosis.

However:

> If a patient who lacks capacity asks you not to disclose personal information about their condition or treatment, you should try to persuade them to allow an appropriate person to be involved in the consultation.

If a patient who lacks capacity continues to refuse, you may disclose relevant information to an appropriate person, if you believe that it is in the patient's best interests. Any decision to do so should be recorded in the patient's notes and you should tell the patient before disclosure. As a foundation doctor, you should involve your seniors in such matters. Nevertheless, it is useful to understand GMC guidance on this issue.

Confidentiality issues in children

The GMC publication '0–18 years: guidance for all doctors' states, regarding confidentiality in young people:

Respecting patient confidentiality is an essential part of good care; this applies when the patient is a child or young person as well as when the patient is an adult … The same duties of confidentiality apply when using, sharing or disclosing information about children and young people as about adults.

Therefore, doctors have the same duty of confidentiality to young people as they do to adults. If a child has capacity to consent, this should be obtained before information is shared.

Importantly, regarding the issue of consent in young people, the GMC publication 'Consent: patients and doctors making decisions together' states:

A young person's ability to make decisions depends more on their ability to understand and weigh up options, than on their age. When assessing a young person's capacity to make decisions, you should bear in mind that:

a. *A young person under 16 may have capacity to make decisions, depending on their maturity and ability to understand what is involved.*
b. *At 16, a young person can be presumed to have capacity to make most decisions about their treatment and care.*

The Family Law Reform Act 1969 affords those who are 16 years or above with the same legal ability to consent to treatment as anyone above 18 years, without the need for consent from a parent or guardian. However, this does not mean that they have the right to refuse treatment. Refusal of treatment in those that are under the age of 18 years with capacity is permitted provided that there is one consenting parent or guardian, even if the other disagrees.

Furthermore, 'Gillick competence' refers to a child who is under the age of 16 years who is deemed able to consent, as they have demonstrated 'a sufficient understanding and intelligence to be capable of making up their mind on the matter requiring decision', without the need for parental consent.

With young people that lack capacity, consent should be obtained from a parent. If the parents cannot agree, and this cannot be resolved informally, it may be necessary to seek legal advice about whether an application should be made to the court.

The issue of confidentiality and consent in young people is a complex area. Discussion with seniors is recommended when issues arise while providing care for young people, particularly regarding treatment without parental knowledge and refusal of treatment.

Confidentiality issues and driving

It is the duty of the licence holder to notify the DVLA if they have a medical condition that may affect their ability to drive.

Supplementary guidance issued by the GMC in 'Confidentiality: reporting concerns about patients to the DVLA or the DVA' states:

> If a patient continues to drive when they may not be fit to do so, you should make every reasonable effort to persuade them to stop. As long as the patient agrees, you may discuss your concerns with their relatives, friends or carers … If you do not persuade the patient to stop driving, or you discover that they are continuing to drive against your advice, you should contact the DVLA.

A patient is therefore responsible for informing the DVLA if they are medically unfit to drive. You should explain to the patient that their condition may affect their ability to drive and that they have a legal duty to inform the DVLA. Alternatively, if a patient is not able to understand the advice you have given them, you should inform the DVLA immediately.

If a patient continues to drive against medical advice, and every effort has been made to persuade them to stop, you must inform the DVLA. You should also inform the patient that a disclosure has been made. It is the legal responsibility of the DVLA to decide if an individual is medically unfit to drive.

Breaking confidentiality
There are instances where you may have to disclose confidential information. The main reasons for disclosure are:

1. Where the patient has consented to disclosure
2. Where it is in the public interest – to protect individuals or society from risk of serious harm, including serious crime or suspected or known communicable disease
3. Where there is a court order by a judge or presiding officer.

The GMC advises that the patient should be informed that a disclosure will be made even if consent has not been sought, unless it is impracticable to do so, where this would put yourself or others at risk of serious harm or undermine the purpose of disclosure.

In instances where you consider disclosing confidential information without consent, you must weigh the harm to the patient and doctor–patient relationship against the benefits which result from the release of this information.

EXAMPLE 4

You are on the ward when a patient reports her expensive bracelet is missing. Towards the end of your shift you enter the staff room to retrieve your bag, when you collide with a colleague. You notice an expensive bracelet on her wrist similar to the one that went missing.

Rank in order the following actions in response to this situation (1 = Most appropriate; 5 = Least appropriate).

A Call the police so that they can investigate further.

B Tell the patient that her bracelet has been found in the staff room.

C Discuss with your colleague what has just happened in order to determine whether she indeed stole the bracelet.

D Ask your colleague if she stole the bracelet.

E Tell your consultant immediately.

Approach to question

This scenario poses a dilemma; you must act on what you have seen, while handling the situation carefully so as not to severely affect your professional relationship with your colleague. You should therefore deal with the situation in a sensitive manner in order to elicit more details from your colleague (Option C). This is clearly the most appropriate response.

Involving a senior (Option E) may seem overly drastic, but allows for the matter to be investigated further and is more appropriate than accusing your colleague (Option D) and thereby compromising your professional relationship with them. Option E is therefore preferred to Option D.

Telling the patient that the bracelet has been found (Option B) would not be appropriate since this has not been confirmed. It also does not allow for your colleague to explain herself and may compromise the patient's trust in the healthcare team. Given that there is no active dispute requiring mediation, or definitive evidence that the patient's possession was stolen, the least appropriate response would be to call the police (Option A). Furthermore, such action may compromise your professional relationship with your colleague.

Example 4 answer is: C, E, D, B, A.

Guidance on Example 4: Breaking the law

In these scenarios, responses which allow you to establish facts should be placed ahead of options which relate to preventative measures or accusing colleagues. You will also need to assess the severity of the offence to determine whether more senior authorities need to be involved, and act accordingly.

As with all the questions you encounter, you must also assess whether patient safety is compromised. If this is the case, you would need to take action to protect patients, and inform your seniors. With more severe offences which would require the involvement of the police, as a foundation doctor it would be more appropriate to discuss the case with your seniors before proceeding.

See Example 2 for GMC guidance on the conduct and performance of colleagues.

EXAMPLE 5

You are approaching the end of a long shift. You have arranged to meet some friends but you are already running late. Your colleague, who is supposed to be taking over, has still not arrived on the ward for you to hand over.

Choose the THREE most appropriate actions to take in this situation.

A Check with medical staffing to ensure your colleague has not called in sick.

B Hand over to the registrar who has just started his shift if he is willing to accept the responsibility.

C Instruct the nurses to tell your colleague to call you when he arrives for the handover and leave the ward.

D Tell your consultant that your colleague was late and it resulted in you staying unnecessarily.

E Call your colleague to determine why he is delayed.

F Cover the shift until your colleague arrives and offer to stay for the entire shift if your colleague is indeed unwell.

G Leave when your shift ends as you have made a commitment to your friends.

H Leave a detailed handover sheet on the ward.

Approach to question

This question asks for the three most appropriate responses. You must make patient safety your priority and responses which would result in inadequate cover are therefore not suitable (Options C, G and H). These options would result in there being no doctor to cover the patients that you are looking after.

It would be sensible to determine why your colleague has not arrived (Option E) and check that he is not unwell (Option A), as this would allow alternative arrangements to be made. You have just completed an entire shift so it would be inappropriate to work another one (Option F), as you will be tired and this is likely to impact on the care of your patients. Telling your consultant (Option D) would not deal with the problem and will impact on your working relationship with your colleague. You should establish the facts behind why your colleague has not arrived before deciding to escalate the issue. Informing the consultant is therefore an inappropriate response. Considering the circumstances and the remaining options, informing the registrar who has just started their shift (Option B) is acceptable as it would enable adequate cover of patients by another doctor. While this is not ideal, this is the best available option. It is important to note that the registrar is suitably qualified to provide cover for you. However, the converse is not true and should the registrar find himself in this scenario, he would have to remain at work until a suitably qualified doctor was available to take over.

Once you have chosen the best three responses, perform a final check to ensure that they are all appropriate and do not contradict one another. The three options which have been selected would be most suitable given the options available.

Example 5 answer is: A, B, E.

Guidance on Example 5: Work/life balance

With these questions, you must consider whether patient safety is at risk. The GMC publication 'Good Medical Practice' states that 'Good doctors make the care of their patients their first concern'. You have a duty to ensure that there is appropriate cover for patients. The same GMC publication states:

> You must be satisfied that, when you are off duty, suitable arrangements have been made for your patients' medical care. These arrangements should include effective hand-over procedures, involving clear communication with healthcare colleagues. If you are concerned that the arrangements are not suitable, you should take steps to safeguard patient care.

There are usually options in the question which allow for a compromise: providing cover for patients, while allowing you to attend to your commitments outside of the hospital. Working excessively is not sustainable and will impact on patient care if you are tired and having to cover shifts you have not been scheduled to do. However, it is worth noting that when adequate cover from a suitably qualified doctor has not been arranged, it is better for patient welfare that you remain at work rather than having no cover available at all. In this instance, it would be acceptable to continue working until a suitable person arrives to replace you, despite the risk of mishap in your tired state. As a foundation doctor, when you have an excessive workload you may be able to deal with this by prioritising urgent tasks and delegating other jobs to those who are suitably qualified to carry them out.

You may also encounter questions which relate to gifts or payment for the work you do. You must assess whether the gift offered is appropriate for the level of care or service provided. Wholly inappropriate gifts should be declined. Declining such a gift may offend the patient and adversely affect your relationship with them. However, patients need to be made aware that they are not obliged to reward your services and assured that not doing so will not impact on the quality of the care that they receive. The GMC publication 'Good Medical Practice' states:

> You must be honest and open in any financial arrangements with patients. In particular: … you must not encourage patients to give, lend or bequeath money or gifts that will directly or indirectly benefit you.

If the gift is disproportional to the service that was offered, it may be more appropriate to politely decline the gift and sensitively explain to the patient why you are doing so. Practice questions related to this topic are available in Chapter 5.

SUMMARY

These examples highlight the important and popular underlying themes in many SJT questions. As you work through the questions in this book, it will become apparent that your priorities in these scenarios are the same.

Firstly, you should endeavour to deal with the matter at hand <u>directly</u> and as <u>decisively</u> as possible. This should be while <u>minimising potential damage</u> to <u>working relationships</u> where possible. Where <u>patient</u> safety becomes a consideration, you must ensure that it is not compromised and that it <u>supersedes</u> other issues. Dilemmas may arise where patient safety comes into conflict with professionalism. In instances where this does occur, your duty to protect patients must come first, even at the expense of your working relationship with a colleague. Therefore, if a colleague's ability to work is compromised due to personal problems or lack of competence, then you must take action to safeguard patients. Once the immediate situation is dealt with, preventative strategies, such as the use of incident forms, may then be employed. Options which are in clear breach of GMC guidance, including those that compromise patient safety or breach confidentiality, should be ranked below all other options in accordance with the severity of the infringement. This advice is extracted from the principles outlined by the GMC in the wide-spanning guidance provided by their publications. However, the guidance that has been produced is not completely comprehensive and given the impossibility of foreseeing every possible scenario, it is necessary to continue extracting such principles and remaining sufficiently flexible to employ them appropriately.

With this in mind, it is worth spending time to review 'Good Medical Practice', 'Confidentiality' and the guidance on consent. When approaching these publications, it is inadvisable to memorise the specifics, rather you should identify the ethical influences and morality of the actions that the GMC advises. Extracting these details will better equip you for the unanticipated scenarios which may arise in the SJT questions, and will help you to analyse the questions with the correct priorities in mind, especially in cases where best practice is not represented in the available options. Greater clinical experience and practice questions will further exercise your ability to apply the relevant principles and manage these challenging situations appropriately.

4: Procedures and Protocols

INTRODUCTION

Starting your working career as a doctor involves a steep learning curve, where you must become accustomed to the various procedures and protocols that exist within the clinical environment. A knowledge and appreciation of this will allow for a smoother transition into this new role. It will also be of benefit when tackling SJT questions, as you will have a greater understanding of your priorities and of the challenges involved in the effective delivery of healthcare.

This chapter is intended to inform readers of the mechanisms existing within hospitals and the Foundation Programme, which are helpful to have an awareness of when starting work as a foundation doctor. Knowledge of the topics included in this chapter will also be of benefit in tackling SJT questions.

FOUNDATION DOCTOR: TRAINING

Overview

It is vital that you continue to develop your skills and knowledge base following qualification as a doctor. Evidence of your achievements and assessments can be recorded electronically on the e-Portfolio. In addition, regular meetings with your supervisors ensure that you set challenging yet achievable targets and continue to develop over the course of the year.

Clinical supervisors

As you move through each placement, you are assigned a different clinical supervisor. This consultant is responsible for your progress and development during the placement. Normally, the clinical supervisor is also the consultant responsible for your team, although this may vary between Foundation Schools. They ensure that your record during the placement is satisfactory and complete a report at the end of your placement with assistance from a supervision group consisting of other colleagues, including therapists and nurses, with whom you work.

Educational supervisors

The educational supervisor stays with you over the course of the year. They are responsible for reviewing your targets at the start of each placement, and ensuring that they have been met at the end. They are also involved in providing the recommendation for the end-of-year sign-off to the responsible local panel, which confirms satisfactory completion of the foundation year 1 (FY1) placement.

The e-Portfolio

The e-Portfolio is an electronic logbook which exists to record your skills and achievements over the course of the year. It is also a record of the supervised learning events that you have completed. These can be reviewed at meetings with your clinical and/or educational supervisor and at the end-of-year sign-off to ensure that you have fulfilled the requirements of the foundation curriculum. Personal reflections can be recorded on the system, which provide an opportunity for you to share significant encounters with patients and other members of the healthcare team. These can also be discussed with the educational supervisors at the allocated meetings and linked to sections of the foundation curriculum as evidence of achieving the required competencies.

FOUNDATION DOCTOR: DOCUMENTATION

Overview

Accurate and reliable note-keeping is an important aspect of patient care. Proper documentation ensures that a permanent record of events is maintained and is accessible to other members of the healthcare team, promoting better patient care and communication. Following an adverse event, the patient's medical notes may prove to be the only defence that a certain action was performed or that a differential diagnosis was considered. With this in mind, it is important to be meticulous when writing entries in the notes, ensuring that they are accurately dated with the time stated. Signatures should be legible or otherwise names printed with a bleep number documented.

Other forms of documentation that may be required include fit notes, incident forms and drug charts. Regardless of the type of document to be completed, it is essential that, in accordance with General Medical Council (GMC) guidance:

> You must be honest and trustworthy when writing reports, and when completing or signing forms, reports and other documents.

Fit notes

Fit notes may be issued where patients are deemed unfit to work, or potentially fit for work if adequate arrangements are made. The form contains a box for each of these criteria, which is completed by the doctor and issued to the patient. Specific details regarding the patient's condition should be avoided to protect confidentiality. It is generally adequate to state generic details outlining the patient's reason for admission and these are more likely to be acceptable to patients.

The maximum period of time a fit note can be issued for, for an inpatient, is generally two weeks, with any extension having to be reassessed by the patient's GP. Patients should otherwise self-certify for periods of sickness up to one week, and should not require further documentary evidence.

Incident forms

A clinical incident is any adverse event or near miss involving patients, and includes drug errors, injury to patients, and complaints. Incident forms are used to highlight these errors so they can be investigated thoroughly in order to uncover an underlying cause and implement measures to prevent recurrence. In the event of a clinical incident, measures should be taken to correct the error to limit the impact upon patients. Incident forms should be completed, ideally within 24 hours to preserve the quality of the information, and submitted to the department responsible for risk management.

Some incidents may only become apparent after a delay, and these too must be reported in a timely manner on discovery of the errors which have occurred. Incidents are investigated internally following the collation of information, with external bodies notified if appropriate. The level to which incidents are investigated is governed by the seriousness of the event. Important aspects of the incident are considered, particularly the impact on the affected person, the potential harm that could have occurred and the risk of recurrence.

The most in-depth investigations are reserved for the most serious incidents, and this involves a root-cause analysis. This is where the events are examined thoroughly with a view to exposing the fundamental causes of the incident. The process may include interviewing the parties involved or reviewing patient records. Once the cause is identified, appropriate mechanisms are assessed and employed to prevent repeat incidents. After a period of time, the measures are reassessed to monitor the efficacy of the intervention, and this process is known as 'closing the loop'.

Prescribing and community prescriptions

You must ensure that the prescriptions that you write are safe and accurate, ensuring that you are aware of the patient's allergies and past medical history. FY1s are able to prescribe for inpatients and on their discharge. While prescribing under supervision is permitted, they cannot self-prescribe, or independently write private or community prescriptions (FP10s). It is also stated that FY1s should not prescribe or administer cytotoxic drugs or immunosuppressants, with the exception of corticosteroids.

On progression to FY2, doctors achieve greater prescribing rights, as well as the authority to independently discharge patients and to self-prescribe, although this is not recommended. Supplementary guidance offered by the GMC states that:

> *Objectivity is essential in providing good care; independent medical care should be sought whenever you or someone with whom you have a close personal relationship requires prescription medicines.*

This means that this additional privilege should be exercised with caution and avoided where possible.

DEATH AND DYING

Overview
Taking care of dying patients is an important aspect of practice as a foundation trainee. Care does not end when a patient dies, and your duty to protect confidentiality in addition to acting in a patient's best interests continues beyond their passing. These cases often present challenging dilemmas that involve not only the patient, but also their relatives.

When a patient's condition is identified as terminal, difficult decisions may need addressing. Questions may be raised about whether the patient will benefit from cardiopulmonary resuscitation (CPR) or if it is appropriate to stop active management and focus on supportive treatment with the aim of promoting the patient's comfort in their final moments.

Do Not Attempt Resuscitation (DNAR) forms
The resuscitation status of a patient should be considered at the time of admission and made by the most senior admitting doctor. Resuscitation status applies to the current admission only, and should be reassessed on subsequent admissions. As the clinical condition of the patient changes, there should be no hesitation in reviewing the prior decision and either cancelling or invoking a DNAR order.

The DNAR form is an active decision that is taken to withhold CPR only. The success rates of CPR are highly variable, with some estimates suggesting that 20 per cent of patients who have had a cardiac arrest as inpatients survive to hospital discharge. A decision to complete a DNAR form for a patient is taken where CPR is likely to be futile or will result in a poor outcome. In this way, it may help to protect particular patients from a distressing and undignified death. However, the presence of a completed DNAR form does not mean a patient's condition should be considered terminal – they may well go on to be discharged from hospital following successful treatment. In addition, it should not affect treatments, such as the administration of fluids, nutrition, oxygen or antibiotics, which should be continued.

DNAR forms: Patients with capacity
A doctor may implement a DNAR form when a medical judgement, based on the clinical condition and co-morbidities of a patient, suggests that CPR is unlikely to be successful. Such a decision requires significant experience

and should not be undertaken lightly. In these cases, such a decision does not legally require consent from the patient or relatives. It is, however, advisable to involve patients in the decision-making process.

In instances where post-resuscitation quality of life is questioned, a discussion should be instigated with the patient on the subject. This conversation should preferably be led by a senior doctor and should focus on the patient's views. The outcome of the discussion should be an informed decision made by the patient.

DNAR forms: Patients without capacity

In cases where the patient lacks capacity as determined by the Mental Capacity Act 2007, and CPR is judged unlikely to be successful, the situation should be dealt with in the same way as in cases where the patient possesses capacity. Once again, this is a clinical judgement that does not require consent from the patient or their relatives, but you should aim to involve them in this discussion.

Where questions are raised regarding the quality of life in such a patient, the matter should be dealt with in accordance with the guidance on capacity covered in the previous chapter. In essence, the patient should be fully assessed for capacity and if it is determined to be compromised, the doctor should act in the patient's best interests. When determining best interests, it is wise to consult relatives who know the patient well to gain an insight into their pre-morbid thoughts and wishes concerning resuscitation.

Advance directives

Some people may elect to outline specific instructions and requests in a legal document which may be applied in the future when, as a patient, their capacity to make decisions becomes diminished. These documents can only be made by a person who currently has capacity and is over the age of 18. Given the potential dilemmas that may arise from such a document, additional strict criteria must be met. This includes that the request must be in writing, signed by the individual and witnessed by another who also possesses capacity. Furthermore, the directive must be specific to the current situation in order to be valid.

Advance directives may apply to terminal care, such as CPR, and may specify refusal for life-saving interventions. In such instances, an explicit statement must be made confirming that the decision applies 'even if life is at risk'. In the absence of such a statement, it cannot apply to life-sustaining treatment. Advance directives should be adhered to, however, it is important to note that, in the presence of an advance directive with doubt about its validity, it is acceptable to act in the patient's best interests to sustain life until the validity can be clarified.

The Liverpool Care Pathway

In the final moments of life, the healthcare team may act to ensure that the patient is comfortable and the salient problems affecting them are addressed. The Liverpool Care Pathway (LCP) is an accepted framework to standardise practice regardless of the patient's environment in the days and hours preceding death. It refers to adequate symptom control, for example treating agitation with sedation or nausea and vomiting with anti-emetics.

It is important to note that this not only applies to patients with cancer, but to all patients who are recognised as being in the final phase of their life. The Palliative Care team can provide advice on appropriate drugs and the discontinuation of those which are unnecessary. The aim is to help patients die with dignity and to avoid unnecessary distress. If the clinical condition of a patient were to improve, the LCP may be discontinued if appropriate.

Reporting cases to the coroner

It is possible to discuss cases with the coroner's office in instances where there are complex issues surrounding a patient's death. In general, these are suspicious and uncertain cases, and they include:

1. Sudden, unexpected or unnatural cause of death
2. Cause of death unknown
3. Death within 24 hours of hospital admission
4. Not being seen by a doctor within 14 days of death
5. Surgery- and anaesthesia-related death
6. Drug- and alcohol-related death
7. Doubtful stillbirth
8. Death in prison
9. Domestic and industrial accidents.

When a death is reported, the coroner may request that a pathologist examines the body of the deceased to carry out a post-mortem examination. Alternatively, they may be able to offer suggestions regarding the cause of death which may be used to allow for a Medical Certificate of the Cause of Death (MCCD) to be issued.

Confirmation of death and certification

When notified of a suspicion that a patient has died, it is important to attend without any unnecessary delay. Death must be confirmed by a doctor performing a thorough examination. Specifically, the following criteria must be met.

The patient must demonstrate:

1. Unresponsiveness to pain stimulus
2. Absent pupillary reflexes
3. Absent central pulses (carotid and femoral pulse)
4. Absent heart sounds
5. Absent lung sounds.

It is also advisable at this point to check for any pacemakers, which must be removed prior to cremation.

Following the confirmation of death, it is important to ensure accurate documentation in the notes. This should include the time of death and the particulars of the examination performed.

You may also be required to complete an MCCD for the deceased patient. This is a certificate that is completed by the doctor specifying the time and cause of death. It should only be completed when a cause of death is known, otherwise a discussion with the coroner's office may be required. The particulars of this are discussed below.

The cause of death is recorded on the MCCD within an individual box. Abbreviations must not be used, and specific conditions should be mentioned as opposed to the mode of death. The cause of death is separated out further into 1a, 1b, 1c and 2 subsections. It is not mandatory to have an entry in each subsection, with the exception of 1a, the primary cause of death, which must be completed. The condition stated in 1c should lead to that in 1b, which in turn should lead to 1a, the primary cause of death. The remaining co-morbidities may be listed in section 2, if they contributed to the death but did not directly lead to death. An example of this would be as follows:

1a. Pulmonary oedema
1b. Myocardial infarction
1c. Hypercholesterolaemia
2. Hypertension, type 2 diabetes mellitus

The bereavement team at the hospital will be available to provide guidance throughout this process, and is responsible for liaising with the family of the deceased and providing them with further information on registering the death.

INVESTIGATIONS

Overview

Investigations should be carefully selected to help confirm a diagnosis after eliciting a history and thoroughly examining a patient. The drawbacks of each investigation should be balanced against the benefits, and where the outcome is unfavourable, alternative options should be sought. When in doubt, a senior should be consulted to advise on the necessary tests and the justifications for them.

While appearing harmless, inappropriate selection of blood tests may impact on the level of care a patient receives. For instance daily blood tests on a patient that is clinically well may result in treatment of numbers rather than the patient. Some investigations may require vetting from a radiologist where the case must be defended before them in order to ensure that it is clinically indicated and does not expose the patient to unnecessary radiation. Before undertaking this, it is important to have an appreciation of the case that is to be made.

Blood: 'Group and save' vs. crossmatch

Blood that is collected for the purposes of administering a transfusion must be obtained observing strict protocols. The purpose of this is to avoid clinical mishaps where a patient's identity is confused with that of another. As such, it is important that the details on the blood sample are completed by hand, at the patient's bedside following verbal confirmation of their identity or their wristband when this is not possible. The details on the bottle should match those on the form.

When selecting the service required, an assessment of the patient's need should be made. In non-urgent cases where there is doubt as to whether blood products will be required, a 'group and save' should be requested. The sample blood is then grouped (ABO), and preserved in case blood products are required at a later time, when the sample will be used for a retrospective crossmatch. A 'group and save' is also useful when blood is needed immediately, as transfusion products can be supplied faster than with a crossmatch. A crossmatch involves a sample of the donor and recipient blood being mixed and analysed for a reaction, which is a process that takes at least 45 minutes. Crossmatched blood should be requested when a known volume of blood will be required at a specific time, an example being during elective surgery where blood loss is anticipated. In other instances a 'group and save' may suffice, where surgery is low risk and significant blood loss is not expected. Whenever a blood transfusion occurs, a crossmatch is always performed to ensure the patient's safety; the only variable is the time at which it is performed. In emergencies, the test is performed in retrospect after or at the time of the transfusion in order to minimise the delay in the critically unwell patient receiving their transfusion. In elective cases, the crossmatch is performed in advance, given that there is no need for the patient to receive the blood quickly.

Imaging

The 'Ionising Radiation (Medical Exposure) Regulations 2000' (IR(ME)R) state that:

> *All medical exposures to ionising radiation must be justified prior to the exposure being made.*

Therefore, careful consideration must be made before an investigation is requested.

Given that some modes of imaging do not expose the patient to radiation, such as ultrasounds and unenhanced magnetic resonance imaging (MRIs), there is smaller argument for harm to the patient. However, these scans are viewed as commodities and thus must be justified in light of their cost and pressure on the scanners from more urgent cases. Computed tomography (CT) scans and x-rays do, however, carry the risks associated with radiation exposure, and must be justified specifically against the harm caused. A chest CT, for example, is equivalent to 70 chest x-rays and therefore its use must be clinically indicated.

When selecting the most appropriate scan, other factors such as the probability of visualising pathology and the ability of the patient to tolerate the procedure must be taken into account. For instance, while an MRI of the lumbar spine will provide the best-quality images for analysis, if a patient is unable to withstand the noise or confines of the scanner, the loss in image quality may mean that a lumbar x-ray is a better mode of investigation despite the additional radiation exposure.

SUMMARY

An understanding of the procedures and protocols that exist within the clinical environment will improve the efficiency with which you work. It will also assist you in tackling ethical dilemmas that may arise and in answering SJT questions, by having a greater appreciation of what is feasible and appropriate when presented with various scenarios.

Other protocols do exist which have not been covered, such as patient referrals, ordering of special tests and appropriate antibiotic selection. Such details vary considerably between hospitals, and further information on this, as well as the topics covered in this chapter, can be obtained at a local level.

5: Practice Questions

Question 1

You are looking after a patient who is a long-standing smoker and presented with weight loss and haemoptysis. Initial investigations are strongly suggestive of lung cancer. On your way to another ward, the patient calls you over and asks you directly if he has cancer.

Rank in order the following actions in response to this situation (1 = Most appropriate; 5 = Least appropriate).

A Arrange to have a discussion with the patient in a quiet room with a senior nurse, handing your bleep to a colleague.

B Explain to the patient that you are awaiting the results of investigations, but you will discuss the findings as soon as you can.

C Reassure the patient that he has nothing to worry about.

D Tell the patient that you will chase up the results of the investigations, and request that one of your senior colleagues discuss these with him.

E Explain to the patient that it is likely he has cancer.

Question 2

You are an FY1 on a medical firm. You walk into the treatment room ahead of the morning ward round to find a staff nurse putting some medicines from the cabinet into her pocket. You suspect that she is self-medicating.

Rank in order the following actions in response to this situation (1 = Most appropriate; 5 = Least appropriate).

A You ask to speak to the nurse in a private setting and request that she does not continue to work today.

B You arrange to speak to your consultant at the end of the ward round.

C You ignore what happened as you do not want it to affect your working relationship with her.

D You inform the Nursing and Midwifery Council (NMC) of the event.

E You immediately inform the ward sister of the situation.

Question 3

You are an FY1 on an elderly care firm. One of your patients, who is increasingly forgetful with a history of dementia, is visibly distressed after finding that his wallet is missing. He is adamant that one of the nurses is responsible.

Choose the THREE most appropriate actions to take in this situation.

A Fill in an incident form.
B Reassure the patient that he has not lost anything.
C Give the patient appropriate sedation to calm him down.
D Ask the nurses if they are aware of the patient's missing wallet.
E Discuss the issue at the multidisciplinary team meeting later today.
F Ask the patient for a description of what was lost and when it was last seen.
G Contact the police.
H Reassess the patient for worsening of his condition.

Question 4

You are an FY1 on a busy surgical firm. You share the workload with another FY1 colleague who is consistently late for work. This has been going on for the past fortnight.

Choose the THREE most appropriate actions to take in this situation.

A You discuss your colleague with the nurses on the ward to determine whether her actions have compromised patient care.
B You arrange to discuss this with your colleague, where you tell her that this cannot continue.
C You work harder to compensate, as this is unlikely to continue long term.
D You call your colleague's partner to determine whether there are any personal problems.
E It is important that this does not affect your working relationship with her, so you wait for your seniors to notice her poor punctuality.
F You discuss with your seniors what has been happening.
G You speak to other FY1 colleagues for their opinions on how unprofessionally your colleague has been acting.
H You request that your colleague makes up the hours at the end of her shift.

Question 5

You are an FY1 covering a night on-call. You are called to see a patient who has acute delirium and was physically abusive to a nurse on the ward. The patient is trying to self-discharge, despite not being medically fit. The sister on the ward does not feel that this is the most appropriate place for him.

Choose the THREE most appropriate actions to take in this situation.

A Move the patient to a locked ward.
B Request a psychiatric review.
C Sedate the patient as he is trying to leave the ward and disrupting other patients.

D Calm the patient down and assess him.

E Restrain the patient yourself with the help of the nurses so that you can fully assess him.

F Ask security to come and restrain the patient from leaving.

G Allow the patient to discharge as he has clearly informed you of his intention.

H Ask for senior help in managing the patient.

Question 6

One of your patients is very grateful for the care she has received in hospital. Her chronic condition requires frequent short hospital admissions and each time she is discharged she presents you with a bottle of wine. She is again ready for discharge, when she offers you another bottle of wine.

Rank in order the following actions in response to this situation (1 = Most appropriate; 5 = Least appropriate).

A Ask your consultant to politely have a discussion with the patient to tell her that these gifts are not required.

B Decline the gift sensitively and accept it reluctantly if she insists.

C Accept the gift as you have earned it.

D Accept the gift and explain that you have accepted it on behalf of the healthcare team.

E Accept the gift and explore the reasons.

Question 7

You are called to see an elderly patient who is clinically septic and in urgent need of antibiotics. You insert a cannula and prescribe IV Augmentin, which you instruct the nurse to give immediately. On returning to the ward an hour later to review the patient, you see that the patient has deteriorated and the IV antibiotics have not been administered.

Rank in order the following actions in response to this situation (1 = Most appropriate; 5 = Least appropriate).

A Withhold antibiotics and start palliative care.

B Find the nurse you dealt with and ask her why she has not administered the antibiotics.

C Reassess the prescription and administer the antibiotics yourself, despite having never done so before.

D Fill in an incident form.

E Call a senior member of your team for further advice.

Question 8

You are an FY1 covering a night on-call and you are asked to rewrite a patient's drug chart. In the process of doing so, you notice that she has been receiving double her normal dose of Omeprazole for three days due to a drug chart error.

Choose the THREE most appropriate actions to take in this situation.

A Correct the issue and inform a nurse that the matter is resolved.

B Wait for the registrar ward round in the morning to pick up the error, the patient has already taken the medication for the day and changing the chart now will have no effect.

C Fill out an incident form.

D Assess the patient.

E Inform the patient of the mistake immediately.

F Highlight the error in the drug chart and inform the patient's consultant in the morning.

G Call a senior doctor for advice on how to proceed.

H Correct the drug chart and make an entry in the patient's notes for the registrar to read on the morning ward round.

Question 9

You are an FY2 doctor working in A&E. Your next patient is a 15-year-old girl with heavy periods, who has come without her parents. Her haemoglobin is sufficiently low and she will need a blood transfusion in the coming hours. She is clearly intelligent and consents to the transfusion but is adamant that her parents do not find out.

Rank in order the following actions in response to this situation (1 = Most appropriate; 5 = Least appropriate).

A Refuse to transfuse the patient until the parents are present: there may be religious or medical reasons not to transfuse.

B Call the patient's parents without telling her. She cannot consent and may abscond if she finds out.

C Transfuse the patient and discharge according to her wishes.

D Encourage the patient to call her parents, and tell her that you will call them if she refuses.

E Explore the patient's concerns about calling her parents.

Question 10

You are an FY1, going home after a busy and eventful day on the wards. On the train, you realise that have forgotten to prescribe the morning insulin for one of your patients, for whom the dose was changed today. You have tried to call the on-call FY1, but she is not answering her bleep. You are running late to catch a theatre show, for which you have tickets.

Choose the THREE most appropriate actions to take in this situation.

A Call the on-call FY1 again in an hour to prescribe the correct dose of insulin.

B Call the medical registrar on-call to prescribe the insulin.

C Wait until morning to prescribe insulin – you will leave early.

D Get off at the next stop and go back to the hospital, missing the beginning of the show.

E Go to the show and after it has finished, go to the hospital to change the insulin.

F Send the on-call FY1 a text message with the patient's name and hospital number and a message to prescribe the insulin.

G Call the ward and tell them to hold the morning insulin until you get there in the morning.

H Call the ward and tell them to bleep the FY1 for you with the necessary information.

Question 11

You have just started as an FY1 on a busy surgical firm. Your registrar, who you feel should be supporting you, is always in theatre and keeps handing you additional work to maximise his theatre time.

Rank in order the following actions in response to this situation (1 = Most appropriate; 5 = Least appropriate).

A Call your registrar and demand that they leave theatre to help you.

B Request to speak to the registrar regarding how you feel and discuss how things could be improved.

C Speak to another surgical FY1 about the situation.

D Make a complaint to the GMC about the situation.

E Speak to your consultant about the situation.

Question 12

There have been a large number of weekend admissions. During the ward round at the start of the week, your consultant has decided to discharge a number of these patients. You return to the ward to complete the discharge paperwork for an elderly patient who had been admitted following a fall. You strongly feel she would need a social package to be implemented before discharge can be considered.

Choose the THREE most appropriate actions to take in this situation.

A Respect your consultant's decision and discharge the patient.

B Discuss with your seniors the need for a social package for this patient.

C Show initiative by contacting social services and occupational therapists directly.

D Discuss the case with your registrar, who was absent from the ward round.

E Discuss the case with the nurses on the ward and take their advice.

F Discharge the patient and arrange a social worker assessment in the community.

G Discharge the patient and arrange for her GP to review the need for a social package.

H Ask the physiotherapists to assess the patient before discharge.

Question 13

You are called to see an elderly patient on the ward with a non-productive cough. She refuses to have any more treatment. The family that have come to see her put pressure on you and the nursing staff to do what is necessary to treat her.

Rank in order the following actions in response to this situation (1 = Most appropriate; 5 = Least appropriate).

A Respect patient autonomy by not providing any further treatment.
B Perform a Mini-Mental State Examination (MMSE).
C Ask for senior help.
D Placate the family by issuing treatment against the patient's will.
E Only offer minimal supportive treatment to the patient.

Question 14

You are working in a busy general practice. Your next patient wishes to be started on regular low-dose aspirin. You find that he has no risk factors for heart disease, nor does he have any past medical history. You try to explain that there is no need, but he demands that you give him the drug.

Rank in order the following actions in response to this situation (1 = Most appropriate; 5 = Least appropriate).

A Prescribe a short course and reassess him in a fortnight.
B Explain that it is not in his best interest, but allow him to seek a second opinion if he does not agree.
C Refuse to prescribe the drug.
D Prescribe the drug as he is insistent.
E Explore the reasons why he feels the drug is necessary, and explain why he does not need the drug.

Question 15

A new registrar has joined your busy medical team. You become increasingly aware that he is making inappropriate management plans for the patients under your care.

Rank in order the following actions in response to this situation (1 = Most appropriate; 5 = Least appropriate).

A Ask the nursing staff whether they share your concerns.
B Take the registrar aside and convey your concerns.
C Accept your registrar's decisions as he is a senior doctor.
D Report your concerns to your consultant.
E Contact your defence union's confidential helpline.

Question 16

You are an FY1 on a surgical firm. Your registrar is revising for her membership exam and asks you to hold her bleep for the day. She states that the constant bleeps are a distraction and reassures you that she will remain on-site.

Choose the THREE most appropriate actions to take in this situation.

A Accept the bleep and agree to contact the registrar when she is needed.

B Refuse the bleep, as you are not senior enough to hold a registrar's bleep.

C Call your consultant and complain about your registrar's request.

D Suggest your registrar hands her bleep to another registrar.

E Ask your registrar to hand her bleep to the librarian to take messages.

F Tell her to remove the batteries from the bleep.

G Refuse the bleep and ask the nursing staff to contact you wherever possible to limit the disruption to the registrar.

H Accept the bleep, but express that this is not a long-term solution to the dilemma.

Question 17

You are an FY1 on an obstetrics and gynaecology firm. A 17-year-old girl with an 8-week pregnancy comes to see you, asking for an abortion. She insists that her parents are not informed of her pregnancy or attendance.

Choose the THREE most appropriate actions to take in this situation.

A Inform the patient that you will call her parents. She is under age and requires parental guidance.

B Provide an abortion as the patient is able to consent.

C Conduct a capacity assessment to confirm that the patient is able to consent.

D Explore the reasons for the request to have an abortion. There are other options available.

E Refuse the request for an abortion.

F Ask for a senior review.

G Encourage the patient to tell her parents.

H Educate the patient on safe sexual practice.

Question 18

A patient under your care has been assessed by your registrar on the morning ward round as being fit for discharge. When you return to the ward to discharge the patient a nurse expresses concern about the patient and asks you to reassess him. You feel that he is not ready to be discharged.

Rank in order the following actions in response to this situation (1 = Most appropriate; 5 = Least appropriate).

A Keep the patient in overnight.

B Discharge the patient as planned.

C Ask your registrar to reassess the patient.

D Ask another registrar for a second opinion.

E Call your consultant to discuss this case.

Question 19

A young patient who is grateful for your contribution to her care presents you with a thank-you card. You note that she has written her contact details at the bottom and asks that you promise to remain in touch as friends.

Rank in order the following actions in response to this situation (1 = Most appropriate; 5 = Least appropriate).

A Make the promise and call her in two weeks.

B Ask your consultant to intervene in the situation.

C Agree to keep the promise but do not call her.

D Tell her that you will be her friend only if she no longer comes under your care.

E Tell her that a friendship will compromise any future care that you provide her.

Question 20

A young woman with a history of alcoholism, who you have cared for during her time in hospital, confides in you that she is unhappy in her marriage and has been the victim of domestic abuse at the hands of her husband. She asks you what she should do, but she is afraid to betray her husband.

Choose the THREE most appropriate actions to take in this situation.

A Inform the patient about support groups which may be able to assist her in confidence.

B Inform your seniors of this conversation as they may provide invaluable advice.

C Arrange to see the husband to assess whether the patient is telling the truth.

D Inform the police of your findings.

E Advise the patient that she is able to take action by calling the police.

F Do nothing, as you risk further harm to the patient if the husband discovers your involvement.

G Recommend that the patient leaves her husband.

H Speak to the patient's relatives to obtain a collateral history about the alleged violence. This may be a confabulation important to treating her condition.

Question 21

The family of an elderly patient is grateful for your contribution to her care and is keen to present you with an expensive box of chocolates. Your contribution to the care of the patient consisted of taking her blood on one occasion and writing in her notes on the morning ward round.

Choose the THREE most appropriate actions to take in this situation.

A Accept the chocolates graciously, as they are proportionate to the service provided.

B Accept the chocolates on behalf of the team.

C Tell the family that, with regret, it is against policy to accept gifts.

D Ask the nursing staff to accept the gifts on your behalf, as they contributed more to the patient's care.
E Explain to the family that such a gift is not necessary.
F Refuse the gift as the chocolates are expensive and out of proportion for the service.
G Explore the reasons for the family presenting the chocolates.
H Accept the gift on this occasion and tell the family that they should not offer gifts for any future services.

Question 22

You are an FY1 on a respiratory firm. A patient under your care with a chronic lung condition has been assessed as being suitable for home oxygen as he stated on questioning that he had quit smoking. On a subsequent visit you notice a pack of cigarettes in his jacket pocket.

Rank in order the following actions in response to this situation (1 = Most appropriate; 5 = Least appropriate).

A Call the patient's wife and ask her to convince the patient to stop smoking.
B Inform your consultant immediately, as this may be a risk to the patient's health.
C Overlook what you have seen, as you do not want to falsely accuse the patient and damage the relationship you have built with him.
D Immediately act to withdraw his home oxygen as he is at serious risk of harm.
E Ask the patient further questions to understand what you have seen and if your suspicions are correct.

Question 23

A patient you have assessed to have capacity is bleeding profusely and needs an urgent intimate examination. They refuse to be seen by you and request to be seen by a doctor of the same sex. None are immediately available and they are adamant that you do not examine them.

Rank in order the following actions in response to this situation (1 = Most appropriate; 5 = Least appropriate).

A Wait for a suitable doctor to become available.
B Explain to the patient the urgency of the examination, ask to perform the examination again but respect their request if they continue to request to be seen by an alternative doctor.
C Arrange a compromise, suggesting a chaperone of the same sex to be present during the examination.
D Explain to the patient that the examination is urgent, and insist upon examining them quickly even if they decline, since their condition is potentially life-threatening.
E Listen to their request and respect it but inform them that you will carefully monitor them, and proceed with the examination if further deterioration immediately threatens their life.

Question 24

You are an FY1 covering a busy weekend on-call. You are confronted by an angry relative of a patient who is not normally under your care. The relative demands to know what is happening with the patient's care. You have not seen the patient yourself and only know as much as is written in the weekend handover sheet.

Choose the THREE most appropriate actions to take in this situation.

A Speak to the patient to obtain consent before approaching the relative.

B Tell the relative that you are unaware of the management plan but you will speak to the patient and consult the notes to find out and tell her.

C Politely tell the relative to wait until the weekday when the patient's normal doctors will be able to give her an update.

D Ask your Senior House Officer (SHO), who is also on-call, for advice.

E Ask the nurses who know the patient for information before talking to the relative.

F Refuse to give the relative any information.

G Give the relative the information that you have from your handover sheet.

H Call a doctor who usually cares for the patient for some information.

Question 25

A patient has been involved in a serious car accident and needs a blood transfusion in order to save her life, as alternative measures are no longer viable. Her clinical condition is critical and she is unable to consent, being unconscious. Her father, who is a Jehovah's Witness, is adamant that the religious views against the receipt of blood transfusions are respected.

Choose the THREE most appropriate actions to take in this situation.

A Give the blood transfusion immediately regardless of the patient's views as her life is at risk.

B Explore the daughter's religious views by questioning the father further.

C Withhold the transfusion until the patient is able to consent.

D Call your registrar for assistance.

E Call the chaplain to convince the father to permit the transfusion.

F Withhold the blood as the patient holds views against transfusions.

G Give the transfusion as you cannot currently ascertain the patient's views.

H Offer to contact a religious leader of the faith for further advice and support.

Question 26

You examine a businessman who comes in for a medical check-up. You find that his blood pressure is markedly elevated. He insists that you omit this from your report so that his application for health insurance is not refused. He threatens to make a complaint against you if you disagree.

Rank in order the following actions in response to this situation (1 = Most appropriate; 5 = Least appropriate).

A Advise the patient to obtain a second opinion from another doctor.

B Refuse to provide a report at all if you are forced to omit the truth.

C Explain to the patient that he can have a copy of the document before he consents to you sending it.

D Refuse to provide any assistance as you object to working under the threat of a complaint.

E Send the report in its entirety, the patient has consented to the report and has no right to control its content.

Question 27

You see an elderly patient in clinic. He is unhappy with the number of medications he is taking. He admits to frequently forgetting to take them when he is supposed to, and is concerned because he does not know the indications for taking each drug.

Rank in order the following actions in response to this situation (1 = Most appropriate; 5 = Least appropriate).

A Contact his GP's surgery for a list of his current medication.

B Offer to review the patient's medication with him and explain the reasons why he is taking each drug.

C Tell the patient to see his GP.

D Tell the patient that he must take all his medication as directed.

E Write a letter to his GP outlining the content of your conversation and your plan.

Question 28

A young patient under your care has died unexpectedly. Her family are understandably upset. You explain that she will need a post-mortem examination to determine the cause of death. The patient's father refuses, explaining that her body must be buried within 24 hours, to honour her religious views.

Choose the THREE most appropriate actions to take in this situation.

A Ask the father if there is a religious leader that you can contact.

B Tell the father that he has no choice in the matter.

C Attempt to appease the father by trying to arrange a post-mortem within 24 hours.

D Explore the reasons for the father's refusal further.

E Ask the father if there are any other family members who should be present in the discussion.

F Ask your registrar for advice.

G Appease the father by circumventing the need for a post-mortem.

H Speak to the bereavement office about how to proceed further.

Question 29

One of the nurses on your ward confides in you that she may have sustained a needle-stick injury when taking blood from a patient yesterday. She states that she was unaware of the injury at the time, and only noticed it this morning. The patient has since been discharged.

Rank in order the following actions in response to this situation (1 = Most appropriate; 5 = Least appropriate).

A Tell her to encourage the site to bleed immediately.

B Advise her to visit occupational health.

C Phone the patient from whom the blood was taken and ask them to come in urgently.

D Complete an incident form on the event.

E Advise the nurse not to continue exposure-prone procedures.

Question 30

You are on a cardiology firm, where you see an obese 40-year-old lady with previous cardiac history and a significant smoking history. You discuss her modifiable risk factors, when she asks you to arrange for her to be prescribed nicotine patches. You see from her notes that she has tried these previously, but has been poorly compliant and continued to smoke despite using the patches.

Rank in order the following actions in response to this situation (1 = Most appropriate; 5 = Least appropriate).

A Explore alternative therapies, as you deem nicotine replacement to be inappropriate for this patient.

B Comply with the patient's request and arrange for the nicotine patches to be prescribed, but educate the patient on how they should be used.

C Suggest that the patient tries a period of abstinence from smoking before she tries nicotine replacement again.

D Avoid prescribing the patches but emphasise that she should stop smoking.

E Explore the difficulties she has stopping, and the previous problems she has had with the patches.

Question 31

You are asked to cover a shift for a colleague who has called in sick, but are unable to do so as you have already made plans to attend a concert. While waiting outside the venue, you notice the colleague who had reported in sick, waiting in line with friends.

Rank in order the following actions in response to this situation (1 = Most appropriate; 5 = Least appropriate).

A Tell your colleague that his conduct is unacceptable and that you will inform your consultant if it happens again.

B Overlook what you have seen, as your colleague is normally hard-working and this is likely to be an isolated incident.

C Tell your colleague he can buy your silence if he treats you to a meal after the concert.

D Discuss the issue with your team the following day.

E Inform your consultant of what you have seen.

Question 32

Your consultant arrives for the morning ward round looking unkempt and smelling of alcohol. This is the third day in a row that this has happened. Your colleagues on the team do not appear to acknowledge the recent change in your consultant's behaviour.

Rank in order the following actions in response to this situation (1 = Most appropriate; 5 = Least appropriate).

A Ask your fellow junior doctors for advice.

B Approach your consultant in confidence and ask him to address your concerns.

C Ask your colleagues whether they have noticed the consultant's change in appearance.

D Report the consultant to the GMC for neglect of duties.

E Ignore what you have seen: if your senior colleagues are not concerned, you have nothing to fear.

Question 33

You are taking down the fluids you prescribed a pre-operative patient yesterday. You notice that the bag is already unattached and that the fluids expired last year. The bag is completely empty. You are aware that the stock box from which the bag came was opened yesterday.

Rank in order the following actions in response to this situation (1 = Most appropriate; 5 = Least appropriate).

A Complete an incident form about the matter and then tell the patient.

B Tell the patient that she has received expired medication.

C Check the bag against the drug chart.

D Raise the incident with the ward manager immediately.

E Document the incident in the notes and do not tell the patient.

Question 34

You are an FY1 on a medical firm. One of your patients requires a liver biopsy for a suspicious lesion that was found on a recent CT scan. On the day of the procedure, he is found to have an elevated International Normalised Ratio (INR) of 1.5 despite your best efforts to reverse this. The on-call radiologist, who had been scheduled to do the procedure, is angered by the patient not being adequately prepared beforehand and refuses to perform the procedure at all.

Choose the THREE most appropriate actions to take in this situation.

A Report the radiologist to the GMC.

B Approach the radiologist again after the bloods have normalised.

C Interrupt your consultant, who is doing an endoscopy list, to discuss your options.

D Speak to another radiologist about this radiologist's unprofessional behaviour.

E Explain to the radiologist that you have had limited success trying to fix the issue and explore the available options.

F Apologise profusely to the radiologist and plead with him to perform the procedure.

G Find another radiologist to perform the procedure.

H Speak to your registrar about the urgency of the procedure.

Question 35

You are asked to insert an intrauterine device for a patient in a GP practice. You have never done this before and have only seen it being performed on a model. The senior GP who normally supervises your consultations has been called away to an emergency. The patient is already in the consulting room and the equipment made ready.

Choose the THREE most appropriate actions to take in this situation.

A Do not insert the device, but offer the patient an alternative in the interim.

B You have seen this procedure before and are competent in it, thus you can undertake the procedure.

C Call the senior GP and check if he will be back soon.

D Keep the patient in the room waiting – the GP will be back soon.

E Phone the GP and get her to instruct you over the line.

F Do not insert the device – the patient can come back on another day.

G Look for another senior who is both capable and willing to supervise you.

H Speak to the patient and ask whether she is willing to wait for the GP to come back and insert the device.

Question 36

One of your patients has tested positive to HIV following a sexual encounter on a business trip abroad. He is reluctant to tell his wife and you are concerned that he may continue to have unprotected sex with her.

Rank in order the following actions in response to this situation (1 = Most appropriate; 5 = Least appropriate).

A Do nothing: you cannot break confidentiality.
B Inform the patient that he must tell his wife, or you will have to do it for him.
C Call and involve your consultant.
D Tell the patient that you are going to break confidentiality.
E Try to persuade the patient not to have unprotected sex with his wife, or else to tell her.

Question 37

You are in casualty where the next patient you see is a tourist from Asia who speaks limited English. He complains of acute shortness of breath and you learn that he has asthma, but did not bring his inhalers with him on holiday.
Choose the THREE most appropriate actions to take in this situation.

A Refuse to prescribe inhalers as he is not a registered patient.
B Treat the patient and advise him to return if his symptoms worsen or recur.
C Ensure the patient is followed up by his regular doctor on his return home.
D Tell the patient that you cannot treat him because he does not pay tax.
E Tell the patient that he needs to find a private doctor as he is not eligible for treatment on the NHS.
F Treat the patient for his breathlessness and write him an NHS prescription for his inhalers.
G Treat the patient for his breathlessness and do not write him a prescription for his inhalers.
H Ask your registrar for advice on treatment of this patient.

Question 38

You are covering the night on-call. You are bleeped to see a patient who reports being in pain. You review the patient's drug chart and note that she is on strong analgesia, which seems inappropriate for the condition recorded in her notes. You are not convinced further medication is indicated.
Rank in order the following actions in response to this situation (1 = Most appropriate; 5 = Least appropriate).

A Prescribe more analgesia.
B Record in the notes the patient's observations, and recommend a pain team review in the morning.
C Refuse to prescribe any more analgesia.
D Proceed to take a history from the patient.
E Ask for senior help.

Question 39

A 34-year-old motorcyclist is admitted to casualty following a road traffic accident. He has a pelvic fracture with worsening hypotension. You recognise that this is source of his bleeding and determine that he requires a compressive support. You have never fitted this before and require help. Your senior colleagues are all occupied with other emergencies, and your consultant is off-site.

Choose the THREE most appropriate actions to take in this situation.

A Stabilise the patient as best you can until help arrives.

B Call the consultant who is off-site to instruct you over the phone on how to fit the pelvic support.

C Ask one of the nurses to relay a summary of this patient to your senior colleagues.

D Bleep the ward-based orthopaedic team to come and help you immediately.

E Go and see your seniors to inform them of this emergency so that they can prioritise.

F Call the patient's family immediately.

G The patient is imminently going to arrest – call the crash team pre-emptively.

H Remove the patient's trousers and apply the compressive support as best as you can.

Question 40

You are an FY1 on an elderly care firm. You find that one of your patients has iron-deficiency anaemia, and sensitively explain that she will need further investigations to rule out cancer as a potential cause. She initially consents to a colonoscopy but, on the morning of the colonoscopy, refuses to have the procedure.

Rank in order the following actions in response to this situation (1 = Most appropriate; 5 = Least appropriate).

A Phone the patient's family in order to confirm that you are acting in her interests.

B Respect the patient's wishes and cancel the procedure.

C Do a capacity assessment on the patient.

D Ask her whether she understands the consequences of not having the colonoscopy.

E Perform the procedure, the patient previously has consented and no longer has capacity to choose.

Question 41

You have ten minutes remaining of a long weekend on-call. You are handing over to a colleague who is due to start the night shift, when your bleep goes off.

Rank in order the following actions in response to this situation (1 = Most appropriate; 5 = Least appropriate).

A Do not answer the bleep until the end of handover and assess the request.

B Do not answer but ask your colleague to answer it when they start.

C Answer the bleep, and tell whoever it is to bleep the new on-call FY1 in 10 minutes.

D Answer the bleep and deal with the request.

E Answer the bleep and assess the request.

Question 42

You are an FY1 on a respiratory firm. You notice that your consultant frequently deviates from national guidelines and local hospital policy when treating patients. You have concerns that this is impacting upon patient care.

Rank in order the following actions in response to this situation (1 = Most appropriate; 5 = Least appropriate).

A Call the GMC to investigate the consultant's fitness to practise.

B Speak to another respiratory consultant about your concerns.

C Explore the management decisions with the consultant and the reasons behind them.

D Do a literature search on the management choices for the patients.

E Speak to your registrar about the management decisions.

Question 43

You are treating a foreign doctor for pneumonia. He wishes to be treated with particular antibiotics, which are not in accordance with your hospital's policy for treating a local pneumonia. He firmly states that the antibiotics he has requested are used routinely in his native country and have been effective for his condition in the past. He demands that they are prescribed while his sputum is being cultured.

Choose the THREE most appropriate actions to take in this situation.

A Inform the patient that you must follow the guidelines, and that you are not allowed to deviate from them.

B Prescribe both the local policy and the requested antibiotics so that all bases are covered.

C Ask advice from your registrar.

D Prescribe the requested antibiotics as the patient is from another country and his infection will respond to different antibiotics.

E Take a detailed history from the patient including recent travel.

F Explain that you will prescribe according to local policy. If the patient deteriorates, you will follow his instructions.

G Call the microbiologist on-call to ask their advice.

H Explain to the patient that you will not deviate from the guidelines unless you have sufficient evidence from the sputum culture.

Question 44

A mother comes to see you with her son, who suffers from debilitating headaches. His current episode of headaches has ended but his mother remains concerned about the impact this is having and aggressively demands a CT scan. You do not feel a CT scan is indicated.

Rank in order the following actions in response to this situation (1 = Most appropriate; 5 = Least appropriate).

A Discuss with the mother her ideas and concerns with regards to her son.
B Tell the mother that a CT scan is not advisable as the risks of radiation outweigh any value of the scan.
C Write a prescription for analgesia for the patient.
D Document in the notes the reason for not scanning the patient.
E Obtain a history from child and mother, including school progress and development.

Question 45

You are the on-call FY1 for general surgery over the weekend. You are bleeped to see a young woman who had a recent termination of pregnancy, and is complaining of post-operative pain. You are unsympathetic due to your religious views and feel that your judgement is subjective and compromised.

Rank in order the following actions in response to this situation (1 = Most appropriate; 5 = Least appropriate).

A Call the anaesthetist as post-operative pain is best managed by them.
B Go to tell the patient that you cannot treat her objectively given your religious beliefs, and offer to review her symptoms.
C Ignore your bleep and do not go to see the patient, as you are unable to provide her with unbiased, appropriate care.
D See the patient but do not prescribe any analgesia.
E Call the SHO on-call and ask them to take over, given your moral objection to this case.

Question 46

You notice that one of your patients with a penicillin allergy recorded on her drug chart has been prescribed amoxicillin, a penicillin-containing drug. You note that the patient has already received two doses of the drug.

Rank in order the following actions in response to this situation (1 = Most appropriate; 5 = Least appropriate).

A Complete an incident form.
B Stop the drug.
C Review the patient.
D Reprimand the nurse who administered the drug.
E Inform the sister on the ward.

Question 47

Your FY1 colleague confides in you that he is having relationship problems with his long-term partner. He asks for additional time off, but has already used up his permitted annual leave. You would need to cover his workload as well as your own regular work.

Choose the THREE most appropriate actions to take in this situation.

A Give your colleague as much time off as he needs. He would surely do the same for you.
B Tell your colleague to take time off as required, but to limit the time he takes.
C Advise your colleague to call in sick.
D Advise your colleague to involve the other senior members in the team.
E Cover for your colleague given the risk of him having to repeat the FY1 year if he takes off too much time.
F Tell your colleague to inform the consultant in order to arrange a solution.
G Speak to your colleague sympathetically. Ask about the amount of time that he thinks he will need and attempt to arrive at a compromise.
H Tell your colleague that he will need to pay back the time he takes off in return.

Question 48

Your consultant asks to review the grand round presentation you are due to give in two days' time. You stay up late to work on it ahead of your scheduled meeting with him the next afternoon. It is approaching the early hours of the morning and you still have not finished. You have a ward round to attend to in the morning.

Choose the THREE most appropriate actions to take in this situation.

A Complete the presentation that night and call in sick for the morning.
B Tell your consultant that you will be unable to complete the presentation in time.
C Your consultant expects to see the presentation, so stay up to finish as much as you can.
D Go to sleep and work on the presentation in your free time tomorrow.
E Cancel your meeting with your consultant, explaining that you had personal problems to attend to.
F Give your consultant an update on what you have done and when you expect to complete the presentation.
G Ask a colleague to help complete the presentation.
H Ask your consultant for help with the remaining components of the presentation.

Question 49

You are on the morning ward round, where you review the drug chart for one of your patients. You notice that your consultant has prescribed a drug that is commonly used once-weekly, as once-daily. The patient has received several doses already. You are unsure of the reasons behind this and whether it represents a true prescription error.

Rank in order the following actions in response to this situation (1 = Most appropriate; 5 = Least appropriate).

A Leave the prescription unchanged until you can find out from your consultant if this was intentional.

B Ask the nurses whether your consultant has made any recent drug errors.

C Correct the prescription to once-weekly.

D Inform the patient of the error.

E Contact the consultant on his mobile via switchboard to ask about changing the prescription.

Question 50

You are bleeped to see a patient who has a history of sickle cell disease. He is also known to be an intravenous drug user. He appears to be in distress and pleads with you to give him more morphine. He was admitted two days previously with a similar suspected crisis episode.

Rank in order the following actions in response to this situation (1 = Most appropriate; 5 = Least appropriate).

A Rule out any precipitants, including infection.

B Get a haematology review to determine how the patient should be managed and whether analgesia is indicated.

C Prescribe the patient what he requests.

D Take a quick history from the patient and determine whether he has a care plan.

E Do not prescribe any analgesia until you have confirmed that this episode is a true vaso-occlusive crisis.

Question 51

You are an FY1 on a surgical firm. A patient who was admitted with renal colic wishes to make a complaint against the nurse looking after her, and asks you how she should proceed. Despite repeated requests, she states that she was left in intense pain and not given the analgesia you had written up on her drug chart until you came along and ensured that it was given.

Choose the THREE most appropriate actions to take in this situation.

A Convince the patient not to make a complaint.

B Reprimand the nurse for not putting her patients first.

C Escalate the complaint to the sister and avoid completing an incident form.

D Inform the patient of the complaints procedure.

E Tell the nurse to apologise to the patient.

F Ask advice from your registrar.

G Escalate your concerns to the ward manager and complete an incident form.

H Tell the patient that you will deal with the complaint.

Question 52

A young mother comes to see you with her 1-year-old baby boy. She states that he is breathless and developed a persistent cough. She is concerned about the difficulties she has feeding him, and requests a short course of antibiotics to help him get over his infection. You determine that the baby's symptoms have a viral cause.

Choose the THREE most appropriate actions to take in this situation.

A Explore further why the mother requests antibiotics despite your assurances that the illness is viral.

B Prescribe the antibiotics, given that withholding them will adversely affect the mother.

C Ask the mother if everything else at home is ok.

D Prescribe the antibiotics and tell the mother not to use them unless the illness does not resolve in seven days.

E Do not prescribe the patient antibiotics and tell the mother to return if the illness does not resolve in seven days, or if she becomes concerned.

F Do not prescribe antibiotics and tell the mother to attend A&E if the child's condition worsens.

G Do not prescribe antibiotics and assure the mother that the symptoms will resolve in seven to ten days.

H Explain that antibiotics will not help, but offer advice on symptomatic relief.

Question 53

You are an FY1 on a surgical firm. The patients on the operating list have all been consented and your seniors are now in theatre. You are called to see a pre-operative patient who is due to have a transurethral resection of the prostate (TURP) for an enlarged prostate. Theatre staff have called for the patient, but you are informed by the nurses that the patient has changed his mind and does not want the surgery.

Rank in order the following actions in response to this situation (1 = Most appropriate; 5 = Least appropriate).

A Attempt to move the patient to the bottom of the operating list in order to buy time to convince the patient to have the surgery.

B Inform your seniors that the patient no longer wants the surgery.

C Explore the reasons why the patient has changed his mind about having the surgery.

D Remind the patient that he signed the consent forms in the morning, and that it is too late for him to change his mind.
E Reassure the patient that the surgery will not be performed.

Question 54

A young girl is admitted to casualty with severe burns to both hands. Her mother reports that the child obtained the injuries playing in the kitchen when her head was turned. You suspect non-accidental injury.

Rank in order the following actions in response to this situation (1 = Most appropriate; 5 = Least appropriate).

A Contact the on-call paediatrician to discuss the case.
B Document what you have noted and ask the GP to follow up the child within two weeks.
C Confront the mother in the waiting area.
D Call social services straight away.
E Speak to the mother to obtain a complete account of how the injuries were sustained.

Question 55

You are in theatre assisting your consultant who is stitching an abdominal wound. He inadvertently strikes your finger as you help control the bleeding from the incision site. You realise that you have sustained a needle-stick injury as you start bleeding into your sterile glove. The patient that is being operated on is known to be an intravenous drug user, who has in the past been reluctant to provide any blood for screening tests.

Rank in order the following actions in response to this situation (1 = Most appropriate; 5 = Least appropriate).

A Report to occupational health immediately.
B Remove your gloves and encourage the injury to bleed under a tap.
C Take a blood sample from the patient while they are still under general anaesthetic.
D Intentionally bleed into the patient to ensure the patient must also provide a blood sample, given the likelihood he would otherwise refuse.
E Complete an incident form.

Question 56

A patient comes to see you with a magazine article on a new drug that is shown to be highly effective at treating his chronic ulcerative colitis. He has previously tried many other drugs which have failed to control his condition. He asks to be started on the new drug.

Rank in order the following actions in response to this situation (1 = Most appropriate; 5 = Least appropriate).

A Explore the patient's ideas about the new drug and address his current concerns.
B Refuse to prescribe the new drug as it is too expensive.
C Explain that he should continue with his current treatment plan.
D Explain that the drug is unlikely to be beneficial at this stage of his condition but offer alternatives to achieve greater control of his condition.
E Review the limited available evidence regarding the new drug and this patient's condition.

Question 57

You are an FY1 on a surgical firm. A patient is admitted onto your ward for renal colic. On the morning ward round following return of initial investigations, your registrar dismisses the decision made by the admitting team regarding their management. When the patient asks the registrar about his own decisions, he reveals that the admitting team were 'clueless'.

Choose the THREE most appropriate actions to take in this situation.

A Return to the patient after the ward round and apologise for the registrar's comment.
B Return to the patient after the ward round and clarify the registrar's comment, explaining that the admitting team did not have access to the blood results.
C Ask a member of the admitting team about the discrepancies in the two management plans.
D Inform the patient that she can submit a written complaint about the registrar's comments.
E Confront the registrar after the ward round about the comment.
F Inform the consultant about the registrar's comment.
G Ask your SHO about advice on how to proceed.
H Ignore the comment and continue as normal.

Question 58

You are an FY1 on a busy respiratory firm. The final-year medical students in your team are unhappy with the amount of teaching that they receive on the firm. Their exams are only one month away and they state that they would rather spend their time in the library revising.

Rank in order the following actions in response to this situation (1 = Most appropriate; 5 = Least appropriate).

A Offer them teaching.
B Give them time off during the week so that they can revise.
C Speak to the consultant to discuss how this could be addressed.
D Suggest that they shadow another FY1 who may have more time to teach.
E Insist that the ward is the best place for them to prepare for their examinations.

Question 59

You are on-call over the weekend and review a patient who had an appendicectomy the day before. You prescribe strong analgesia, a decision that the nurse looking after the patient disagrees with. She refuses to give the medication to the patient.

Choose the THREE most appropriate actions to take in this situation.

A Ask a senior colleague for advice.
B Threaten the nurse with an incident form.
C Cancel the prescription, as the nurse knows the patient better than you do.
D Arrange to speak to the nurse privately to discuss the incident.
E Document that the nurse declined to give the medication.
F Review the patient again.
G Discuss with the nurse the reasons why she disagrees with the prescription.
H Insist that the nurse gives the medication to the patient.

Question 60

You are an FY1 on a medical rotation. Your consultant on the ward round decides to discharge a patient who had been admitted following an adverse reaction to the chemotherapy that they received two weeks ago. The routine bloods you had requested return in the afternoon showing a rising C-reactive protein (CRP) and falling white cell count which is below the normal range. His observations are stable and he appears clinically well. The bed manager comes onto the ward to demand that the bed is vacated as there are several patients waiting to be admitted from casualty.

Rank in order the following actions in response to this situation (1 = Most appropriate; 5 = Least appropriate).

A Discharge the patient as per the consultant's instructions from that morning.
B Discharge the patient but arrange a GP appointment in two weeks.
C Speak to your registrar about the case and whether it would be appropriate to discharge the patient.
D Keep the patient in hospital overnight to ensure that his condition does not deteriorate.
E Discuss the findings with the patient and the available options.

Question 61

One of the patients under your care has passed away. Your consultant informs you that you should put down bronchopneumonia as the cause of death. You were most intimately involved in the care of the patient and do not agree. Your consultant is now off-site, and you have just been bleeped that the patient's family are at the bereavement office and waiting for you to complete the medical certificate of cause of death.

Rank in order the following actions in response to this situation (1 = Most appropriate; 5 = Least appropriate).

A Complete the death certificate but with what you feel is a more appropriate entry.

B Refuse to complete the death certificate yourself.

C Discuss the case with your registrar.

D Adhere to the decision reached by your consultant.

E Speak to the coroner's office.

Question 62

You are an FY1 in paediatrics. You administer a vaccination for tetanus to one of your young patients and they are subsequently discharged. You later find that the medication you gave had expired a year ago. The nurse who prepared the trolley blames you and threatens to fill an incident form against you.

Choose the THREE most appropriate actions to take in this situation.

A Speak to the ward sister about the nurse's error and unprofessionalism.

B Explain to the parents what has happened but reassure them that it is unlikely that the error will cause any harm.

C Contact the parents at home to explain what has happened and advise that they should return if there are any concerns.

D Contact the parents at home and tell them that they need to return to casualty straight away, without causing undue alarm by specifying the error that has been made.

E Speak to the nurse to discuss the incident and discourage her from completing an incident form.

F Respond to the nurse by stating that you intend to fill an incident form against her.

G Discuss the incident with nurse and ward sister, and ensure an incident form is completed.

H Seek advice from a consultant who happens to be on the ward but is not a member of your team.

Question 63

A patient is admitted for minor elective surgery. He has discussed his admission with his family. Shortly before he is due to go to theatre, the patient informs you that he wishes to be discharged as he has to pick his father up from the airport. There is no reason to suggest that he lacks capacity.

Rank in order the following actions in response to this situation (1 = Most appropriate; 5 = Least appropriate).

A Get in touch with the patient's wife and get her to persuade the patient not to leave.

B Allow the patient to leave, but request that he returns as soon as possible so that his surgery can be done at the end of the list.
C Contact security to prevent the patient from leaving.
D Explain to the patient the risks of leaving without surgery.
E Allow the patient to leave, but request that he sees his GP if there are any problems.

Question 64

A mother comes to see you with her young daughter. The mother reports that her child has developed a rash which is worsening. On further questioning you find that the child has not had her childhood immunisations as her mother has refused them.

Rank in order the following actions in response to this situation (1 = Most appropriate; 5 = Least appropriate).

A Attend to the patient and take measures to ensure that her condition is stabilised.
B Educate the mother on the importance of vaccines and dispel any misconceptions that she might have.
C Tell the mother that her actions were reckless and her child's symptoms are likely related to her susceptibility to pathogens she would otherwise have been protected from.
D Explore the reasons why the child has not received her childhood immunisations.
E Refuse to treat the patient as the symptoms are the result of thoughtless behaviour by her mother.

Question 65

You are an FY1 on a gastroenterology firm. One of your patients has just been diagnosed with liver cancer. A staging CT scan shows that there is the potential for a curative treatment with surgery. The patient wishes to try alternative medicine and declines surgery.

Choose the THREE most appropriate actions to take in this situation.

A Act in the patient's best interests and start initial blood work and assessment for surgery.
B Ensure that the patient is fully aware of the options and the risks of refusing surgery.
C Explain to the patient that she will likely die without surgery.
D Conclude that the patient is likely to lack capacity, secondary to her deteriorating clinical state.
E Tell the patient that alternative medicine therapy will not benefit her condition.
F Elicit further details about the patient's intended alternative remedies.
G Explore the patient's ideas, concerns, expectations and reasons for refusing surgery.
H Call her mother in an attempt to persuade the patient to reconsider surgery.

Question 66

You are an FY1 on an endocrinology firm. One of your patients has poorly controlled diabetes, and her condition continues to deteriorate as she refuses to adhere to the treatment you have advised. She has just had another emergency admission and you see her as she is transferred to your ward.

Rank in order the following actions in response to this situation (1 = Most appropriate; 5 = Least appropriate).

A Stabilise the patient then discharge her without further advice regarding her condition; she is not receptive to the advice you have previously given her.

B Provide her with literature on her condition to reinforce what has been explained.

C Ensure the patient is fully aware of the impact her choices are having on her condition.

D Treat the patient for the emergency and ensure she is followed up.

E Involve the patient's family so that they can help manage her condition.

Question 67

You are an FY1 working on a GP rotation. A patient comes to see you as he plans to go on holiday in Africa. You advise that he will need a number of vaccinations, including some not available on the NHS, to protect against the various communicable diseases which are prevalent in the areas he is visiting. He declines and makes clear that he will not have these done before he leaves the country as they are too expensive.

Rank in order the following actions in response to this situation (1 = Most appropriate; 5 = Least appropriate).

A Offer the vaccinations free on the NHS.

B Offer the patient alternative chemical prophylaxis against malaria and other common parasites.

C Allow the patient to leave without challenging him.

D Give the patient general advice on measures to avoid contracting infective diseases abroad, including diseases for which he has refused vaccination.

E Inform the patient of the signs and symptoms of the common diseases so that he can seek help if he contracts them.

Question 68

You are an FY1 on a geriatrics firm. One of your patients, who has severe dementia and has been admitted from a nursing home, is found to be malnourished and wearing soiled clothing that does not look like it has been changed in days. You suspect that he is not being looked after adequately by his caregivers.

Rank in order the following actions in response to this situation (1 = Most appropriate; 5 = Least appropriate).

A Obtain a collateral history from the nursing home and patient's relatives.
B Do not take any rash action at this stage.
C Contact social services.
D Ask the GP to review the patient on a home visit after discharge.
E Speak to someone senior about your concerns.

Question 69

You meet for lunch with your new registrar, who has just joined the team following a period of absence due to maternity leave. She becomes very emotional and tells you that she is struggling with her job and cannot cope with the demands of the consultant and the rest of the team.

Choose the THREE most appropriate actions to take in this situation.

A Offer to help with her work.
B Suggest that she takes some more time off work.
C Suggest that she discusses these issues with other registrars.
D Advise that she should seek some counselling.
E Speak to the consultant on her behalf.
F Ask other members of the team to be more supportive as she is having difficulties with the job.
G Explore the difficulties your registrar is having.
H Offer to go with your colleague to speak to your consultant.

Question 70

You are covering a night on-call. You walk through the doctors' mess, where you find your colleague who is also on duty with a half-empty bottle of wine beneath the table in front of him. You can smell the alcohol on his breath and clothes.

Rank in order the following actions in response to this situation (1 = Most appropriate; 5 = Least appropriate).

A Report the issue to the GMC, as your colleague is putting patients at risk.
B Discuss with your consultant what you have seen.
C Discuss with other FY1s what you have seen to help you decide what to do.
D Discard the bottle of wine and avoid telling anyone what you have seen.
E Discuss the matter with your colleague in order to understand what you have seen.

Question 71

You arrange a supervised learning event with your clinical supervisor on the ward, where you examine a patient. Your supervisor then proceeds to ask you questions, many of which you are unsure of the answers to. You feel your supervisor was rude and undermined your abilities in front of the patient.

Choose the THREE most appropriate actions to take in this situation.

A Speak to the programme director, as your supervisor's conduct was inappropriate.

B Speak to your clinical supervisor about the experience.

C Allow some time to gather your thoughts before taking any action.

D Apologise to the patient on behalf of your supervisor.

E Do not take any action, as you do not want your supervisor to know that you were upset.

F Reflect on the experience to determine what you could learn from the feedback.

G Discuss with your colleagues the behaviour of your supervisor.

H Avoid asking your clinical supervisor for any further assessments.

Question 72

The mother of one of your close friends becomes ill, and has been admitted to the hospital where you work. You receive a phone call from your friend while you are at work, where he asks if you can find out what is happening with his mother.

Rank in order the following actions in response to this situation (1 = Most appropriate; 5 = Least appropriate).

A You retrieve the patient's notes and give the information to your friend.

B You refuse to provide any information regarding his mother.

C You speak to the consultant responsible for the patient's care, explain the situation and ask her to provide your friend with the information that he has requested.

D You ask for the patient's consent to look at her notes and speak to her son about her care.

E You explain to your friend that it is against Trust policy to conform to his request.

Question 73

Your educational supervisor contacts you to arrange a mid-placement review to assess your e-Portfolio. You have been on a busy placement, and have not kept up to date with your supervised learning events or completed any of the targets you had agreed upon at the start of the rotation.

Rank in order the following actions in response to this situation (1 = Most appropriate; 5 = Least appropriate).

A Swap your on-calls to delay the meeting as much as possible in order to complete the supervised learning events before the appointment.

B Arrange the meeting and tell your supervisor why you have been unable to meet your targets.

C Change the targets you made on e-Portfolio to make them easier to achieve as your educational supervisor is unlikely to notice the change.

D Meet your supervisor and book another meeting with her in two weeks to reassess the progress that you have made.

E Stay back late after work has finished to complete the supervised learning events.

Question 74

You have three medical students attached to your surgical firm. The registrar from another team points out that the dress code of one of your students is inappropriate and asks you to intervene.

Choose the THREE most appropriate actions to take in this situation.

A Informally speak to the medical student about the issue.

B Do nothing, as the medical student is attached to your team and your seniors have not flagged the issue.

C Ask one of the seniors in your team to discuss the issue with her.

D Speak to other FY1s about how you should approach the issue.

E Tell the medical student to change her dress code but avoid specifying the reasons why you are having the discussion.

F Ask the local administrator, who oversees undergraduate education at the hospital, to contact her regarding the issue.

G Tell the registrar that he should contact the medical student himself.

H Politely decline as you do not see anything wrong in the way the student dresses.

Question 75

You are covering a medical on-call when you are bleeped to attend a cardiac arrest. When you reach the ward, CPR has been commenced by the A&E nurse. You pick up the patient's notes, where you find a valid Do Not Attempt Resuscitation (DNAR) form.

Choose the THREE most appropriate actions to take in this situation.

A Take a blood gas sample.

B Take over from the nurse when she tires during chest compressions.

C Continue CPR until the medical registrar arrives.

D Stop CPR immediately, and open the patient's airway.

E Check the patient's pulse.

F Check whether the patient is breathing.

G Check the patient's pupils.

H Stop CPR and leave the patient alone, as per the DNAR form.

Question 76

You are on a medical rotation with a team that includes three other FY1s. You learn that one of the other FY1s has already arranged her annual leave, without consulting any of the other FY1s so that she can go on holiday. Consequently, due to on-call rota scheduling, the scope for the other FY1s to take their leave is significantly limited, in order to ensure that there is appropriate cover for patients.

Rank in order the following actions in response to this situation (1 = Most appropriate; 5 = Least appropriate).

A Change your own on-calls with another FY1 to accommodate annual leave, to limit the effect of the other FY1's actions on your work/life balance.

B Talk to the FY1 who has taken her leave and negotiate with her to take her leave at another time.

C Speak to your consultant about the situation and the fact that the other FY1s cannot take leave.

D Book your leave for the period that you require to be off work.

E Inform the FY1 who has taken her leave that you will not offer her any assistance in future, in retaliation of her inconsiderate actions.

Question 77

You are an FY1 on a surgical firm. Your consultant has asked you to make a radiology request on a busy afternoon ward round. The same request was declined by the on-call consultant radiologist this morning. Your consultant has now gone to theatre where he does not like to be disturbed and you are still unsure of the reasons behind the request.

Rank in order the following actions in response to this situation (1 = Most appropriate; 5 = Least appropriate).

A Omit some of the details of the request so that it is more likely to be accepted.

B Call the consultant in theatre to confirm the details of the request.

C Ask the consultant radiologist to liaise with your consultant in order to understand the request.

D Wait until the next morning's ward round to confirm what to write on the request form.

E Find your registrar to ask him about the justification for the request.

Question 78

You are on a busy medical firm where you frequently find that the team is understaffed. The consultant arrives on the ward to see all the patients, and then leaves you with the jobs so that she can review the patients on the other ward that the team covers. As a result, you feel that there is insufficient support given, that you leave late and that fewer learning opportunities are available, compared to the FY1s on other medical specialities.

Choose the THREE most appropriate actions to take in this situation.

A Continue as you are but seek out further learning opportunities elsewhere, whenever you are free.

B Approach your consultant about your understaffing concerns.

C Find other learning opportunities and complete whatever jobs that you can.

D Finish your jobs and stay back after hours to learn procedures.
E Consult your educational supervisor about the lack of learning opportunities.
F Work harder to compensate for the lack of support.
G Re-examine your contract to ensure that you are being fairly treated, and ask for your hours to be monitored so that you are paid accordingly.
H Complain to the head of department.

Question 79

You start your new rotation on a respiratory firm that has five consultants who rotate on a weekly basis. You learn that your clinical supervisor is the strictest of these consultants, and has a reputation for failing foundation trainees. You have already got off to a bad start and feel that you are in danger of being failed.

Rank in order the following actions in response to this situation (1 = Most appropriate; 5 = Least appropriate).

A Speak to your registrar for advice.
B Arrange your annual leave such that you avoid working at the same time as your clinical supervisor.
C Arrange a mid-rotation review with your clinical supervisor.
D Work harder from now on to compensate.
E Attempt to change your clinical supervisor.

Question 80

You are on an obstetrics and gynaecology firm and assisting your registrar in theatre. You are operating on a 30-year-old woman who has consented to a removal of a troublesome enlarged ovarian cyst. During the operation it becomes apparent that the lesion is likely to be malignant and the safest option would be to remove the entire ovary (oophorectomy). This would be at the expense of reducing her subsequent fertility and the patient has not consented for this. However, removing the lesion alone risks seeding malignant cells in the operative site. The husband is made aware of the situation, while he is in the waiting room.

Rank in order the following actions in response to this situation (1 = Most appropriate; 5 = Least appropriate).

A Continue to assist the registrar in performing an oophorectomy to prevent the tumour from spreading and causing further harm to the patient.
B Suggest that the registrar takes a biopsy of the lesion only and sends it for histology.
C Inform the registrar that he should only perform the procedure for which the patient has consented.
D Speak to the patient's husband to seek his approval to proceed with the oophorectomy.
E Speak to the patient's husband and ask him what he thinks his wife would want.

Question 81

You are an FY1 on a gastroenterology firm. A patient, who underwent a gastroscopy with biopsies having complained of persistent weight loss and epigastric pain, returns to see you for the results. The patient cannot speak English and all communications have previously been made with the aid of his daughter. The daughter tells you at the start of the consultation not to tell her father if the results indicate he has cancer.

Choose the THREE most appropriate actions to take in this situation.

A Explain to the daughter that it is the patient's decision whether he wishes to know the results or not.
B Ignore the daughter's request, as it is the patient's wishes that matter.
C Arrange an independent interpreter.
D Agree not to tell the patient the results of the procedure.
E Ask the patient whether he would like to know the results of the biopsy.
F Tell the patient that his daughter does not wish for him to know the results.
G Ask the daughter to leave the consultation room.
H Inform your consultant what has happened.

Question 82

You are an FY1 on a medical firm. One of your patients, who has been in hospital for the past two weeks, is due to be discharged. He asks for a fit note to be issued and backdated by two additional days prior to admission, as he was also meant to attend a formal examination at work. He states that he visited his GP prior to attending hospital and that his employer requires the dates of the period of illness be stated on his fit note.

Choose the THREE most appropriate actions to take in this situation.

A Fill in the fit note in accordance with the patient's request.
B Fill in the fit note for the period of admission, and request the patient sees his GP to cover the two days prior to admission.
C Refuse to include the dates requested by the patient.
D Determine when his illness started by enquiring further about his presenting problems.
E Ask your registrar's advice before filling in the form.
F Speak to the employer about the patient's illness.
G Contact the GP to confirm that he was ill in the two days prior to admission.
H Objectively assess the likelihood that he is telling the truth, based on his blood results on admission.

Question 83

You are an FY1 on a medical firm, and just covered the last weekend ward cover. When you return to your regular team the following week, you are informed by your SHO one evening that a consultant from the elderly care team attempted to contact you while you attended 'bleep-free' teaching. Your SHO informs you that the elderly care consultant wishes to discuss your management of one of her patients while you were on-call.

Rank in order the following actions in response to this situation (1 = Most appropriate; 5 = Least appropriate).

A Contact the consultant the following morning, once you have completed the jobs for your regular patients.
B Discuss what has happened with your own consultant.
C Contact the elderly care ward straight away to see if the consultant is still in the hospital.
D Speak to the ward sister on the elderly care ward to see if she is aware of what the consultant wanted to discuss.
E Ignore the message, as the work you do for your regular team must take priority.

Question 84

You are in the lunch queue in the staff canteen. Two FY1s in front of you are discussing the management of a patient's condition. You overhear that one is unintentionally giving the other advice that deviates from hospital policy. You are aware that it may be detrimental to the patient.

Rank in order the following actions in response to this situation (1 = Most appropriate; 5 = Least appropriate).

A Tell the SHO taking care of the patient what has transpired.
B Remind them that they are in a public area and should not be discussing patients.
C Advise them both that there is hospital policy on the topic and that deviation from this may be a risk to patient care.
D Approach the two of them individually immediately afterwards to discuss the case and inform them that the information may be inaccurate.
E Proclaim to them both immediately that the information is wrong.

Question 85

An elderly patient with an anxiety disorder is being investigated for headaches. She becomes restless on the ward and tries to leave. The nurses are having a difficult time preventing her from self-discharging and ask you to see her.

Choose the THREE most appropriate actions to take in this situation.

A Call the psychiatry on-call to come and review.
B Call security to restrain the patient.
C Talk to the patient and try to convince her that she should stay.
D Allow the patient to self-discharge.

E Ask the patient to sign a form confirming her decision to discharge against medical advice.

F Implement a doctor's section to prevent the patient from leaving.

G Sedate the patient as she is agitated.

H Tell the patient that she is not allowed to leave.

Question 86

You are an FY1 on a gastroenterology firm. Your FY1 colleague is Afro-Caribbean and goes to consent a patient in order to insert an ascitic drain. As your colleague goes to assemble the necessary equipment, the patient states that he would rather not be treated by him.

Rank in order the following actions in response to this situation (1 = Most appropriate; 5 = Least appropriate).

A Withhold all treatment from the patient.

B Arrange for the procedure to be performed by another colleague.

C Stop your colleague from performing the procedure.

D Explore the patient's views and concerns.

E Explain to the patient that he cannot choose who treats him.

Question 87

You are an FY1 on a medical firm. You are informed that the relatives of a patient who has recently passed away wish to speak to you. They have previously not been involved in the care of the patient and this is the first time you have met them.

Choose the THREE most appropriate actions to take in this situation.

A Explain that the information that you are able to disclose is limited to protect the patient's confidentiality.

B Consult a senior colleague.

C Sensitively explain that you are unable to provide the information they require.

D Ask the ward sister to speak to the relatives.

E Refer the patient to the bereavement office as your involvement with the patient is over.

F Determine what the relatives wish to discuss and their reasons for doing so.

G Tell the relatives that you will arrange for a senior colleague to speak to them.

H Disclose relevant information to the relatives.

Question 88

You are an FY1 on a medical firm. One of your patients, who has a history of alcoholism, is found to have a tooth abscess and is prescribed metronidazole. You explain that he cannot drink while taking the antibiotic because of the adverse reaction it will induce. You are convinced he is unlikely to be compliant, despite his assurances.

Choose the THREE most appropriate actions to take in this situation.

A Specify your advice to the patient on the discharge summary.
B Tell the patient he is responsible for the consequences of drinking alcohol.
C Tell him not to take the antibiotic if he is going to drink.
D Speak to a microbiology consultant about an alternative antibiotic.
E Discharge him on analgesia alone.
F Do not prescribe the metronidazole as it will result in patient harm.
G Tell the patient's wife not to let him drink.
H Discharge the patient with acamprosate (a drug that prevents alcohol dependence).

Question 89

You are an FY1 on an elderly care firm. One of your patients, who is a Jehovah's Witness, has recently received a blood transfusion for symptomatic anaemia and is now well enough to be discharged. He wishes to speak to you and is adamant that the details of the blood transfusion are omitted from the discharge summary to the GP. Upon hearing this, the discharge co-ordinator informs you that you are contracted to the hospital, which will not be paid for the services extended to this patient unless the summary is honestly completed.

Rank in order the following actions in response to this situation (1 = Most appropriate; 5 = Least appropriate).

A Do not include the blood transfusion in the discharge summary, but phone the GP to let them know.
B Follow the patient's request and omit the details.
C Ignore the patient's request and inform him that you have included the details of the blood transfusion.
D Inform your registrar of the event and request advice.
E Explore the patient's reasons for not wanting his GP to learn of the transfusion.

Question 90

You are an FY1 on a medical firm. You go to find your consultant in clinic as you need to get signed off for the end of your placement. As you enter the room you see him with his arm around a female patient.

Rank in order the following actions in response to this situation (1 = Most appropriate; 5 = Least appropriate).

A Request that the patient leaves the room immediately.
B Discuss what you have seen with your registrar who was on the ward with you.

C Notify the GMC of the improper relationship you suspect the consultant is having.

D Ignore what you have seen as there is likely to be a logical explanation and may threaten you getting signed off by the consultant.

E Speak to your consultant once the patient has left to understand what you have seen.

Question 91

You see a middle-aged woman in clinic with bruises over both arms. On further questioning she reveals that her husband is abusive to her and their young son. She does not want the police involved and pleads with you not to tell anyone.

Choose the THREE most appropriate actions to take in this situation.

A Contact the GP to ensure that the case is monitored and acted upon if the patient changes her mind.

B Contact social services, even if the patient does not consent to this.

C Inform the partner that you are aware of the situation and arrange an appointment to see him.

D Do not inform the partner of what you know, and arrange an appointment to see him.

E Speak to a senior colleague about what you have found.

F Provide the patient with details of support groups and domestic violence help lines in case she changes her mind.

G Respect her confidentiality and do not do anything.

H Inform the police.

Question 92

You are at a mess party with your colleagues from work. You overhear a nurse talking to her friends about how she finds one of the FY1s attractive.

Rank in order the following actions in response to this situation (1 = Most appropriate; 5 = Least appropriate).

A Take the nurse to one side and inform her that her behaviour is inappropriate.

B Inform your consultant.

C Tell the group of nurses that their actions are inappropriate.

D Ignore what you have heard and do nothing.

E Inform the ward sister.

Question 93

You are an FY1 on a medical firm. A nurse presents you with a drug chart belonging to a patient that is not normally under your care. The entire drug chart has recently been rewritten, and the nurse points out that one of the analgesics has been omitted. She informs you that the patient is in pain, and you write the analgesic on the drug chart so that the nurse can administer it. You find out from the patient's notes the next day that this medication was deliberately stopped by the patient's regular team.

Rank in order the following actions in response to this situation (1 = Most appropriate; 5 = Least appropriate).

A Review the patient to ensure that they are stable.
B Confront the nurse that asked you to prescribe the drug.
C Inform the patient's regular team of your actions.
D Apologise profusely to the patient.
E Stop the drug immediately.

Question 94

You are an FY1 on a colorectal firm. You are in a pre-assessment clinic, where you are clerking patients who are due to undergo elective surgery next week. The next patient is due to have a complex surgical procedure that you have never heard of. She asks you to tell her what the procedure involves. You do not have access to a computer, and all you have are the patient's notes.

Choose the THREE most appropriate actions to take in this situation.

A Use your existing knowledge to formulate a description of what you expect the procedure to involve.
B Explain to the patient that she can ask the surgeon in the morning of surgery when she has consented.
C Tell the patient that you will leave the consultation to find out what the procedure involves.
D Ensure that the procedure is explained by a senior colleague before the patient leaves.
E Direct the patient to a reliable patient website.
F Tell the patient that you do not know what it involves.
G Use the patient's notes to gain further details regarding the patient's complaint.
H Do not pre-assess the patient on this occasion given that she is unlikely to consent.

Question 95

You are an FY1 on an elderly care medical rotation. You go to see an elderly woman with multiple co-morbidities and no next of kin. She is in considerable discomfort and states that she has a poor quality of life. She asks you to help her die.

Rank in order the following actions in response to this situation (1 = Most appropriate; 5 = Least appropriate).

A Refer the patient to a psychiatrist as she must be depressed.

B Provide her with sufficient medication to result in a fatal overdose if it were consumed.

C Assess the patient for depression.

D Arrange for her medications and fluids to be withheld so that she will die.

E Explain that you cannot help her die, but offer to provide information on options for assisted suicide abroad.

Question 96

You are an FY1 on a GP rotation. An elderly male patient with poorly controlled diabetes comes to see you for a routine check-up. He states that he wishes to observe an upcoming religious festival by fasting over a month period. You attempt to point out that it would be unwise for him to do so, but he is adamant to follow his religious beliefs. You determine that he has capacity.

Choose the THREE most appropriate actions to take in this situation.

A Tell him that if he does fast, not to take any insulin as he risks becoming hypoglycremic.

B Advise him that it is against medical advice for him to fast.

C Phone the community religious leader for advice, while keeping the patient anonymous.

D Ask him what his religion says about him fasting.

E Ask another GP to intervene.

F Modify the insulin regime as best you can to accommodate the fasting.

G Tell him he can fast as long as he checks his blood glucose levels regularly and acts on them.

H Ask him to inform his religious leader about the facts of his specific circumstances to find out what he should be doing.

Question 97

You are about to leave the ward at the end of your shift when a nurse asks for your opinion on an ECG that was performed on a patient with chest pain. Despite your recommendation that she should contact the on-call team, she proceeds to show you the ECG tracing. It shows dynamic changes which are consistent with a new-onset cardiac event.

Rank in order the following actions in response to this situation (1 = Most appropriate; 5 = Least appropriate).

A Berate the nurse for insisting you review the ECG.

B Contact the on-call team.

C Stay behind to further manage the patient.

D Tell the nurse to contact the on-call team and go home.

E Refer the patient for a cardiology review in the morning.

Question 98

The ward sister approaches you to speak to your FY1 colleague, as patients have started to complain about his body odour.

Rank in order the following actions in response to this situation (1 = Most appropriate; 5 = Least appropriate).

A Sensitively explore any problems your FY1 colleague may be experiencing.
B Escalate the issue to the registrar.
C Tell your colleague that the ward sister has informed you that he has a problem with body odour.
D Do nothing as you do not want to offend your colleague.
E Give your colleague some self-care products as a subtle hint.

Question 99

You are an FY1 on a medical firm. Your consultant frequently requests that you run tests for his private practice before attending to your regular duties for the patients you normally look after. He is currently off-site but has messaged you to ask that you perform blood tests and book scans for his private patients immediately.

Choose the THREE most appropriate actions to take in this situation.

A Prioritise your own patients over the tests for the private patients.
B Prioritise both sets of tasks for the private patients and your patients and complete them in order of need.
C Arrange a meeting with your registrar to discuss the matter.
D Arrange a meeting with your educational supervisor to discuss the matter.
E Arrange the tests for the private patients but inform the consultant that you do not accept responsibility for checking the results, as you need to attend to your patients.
F Do not provide care for the private patients as it is not your duty.
G Attend to the private patients' jobs before attending to your patients, as per the instructions.
H Respectfully advise your consultant that you are not responsible for his private patients, given that it may compromise the care for your other patients.

Question 100

You are an FY1 on a surgical firm, where one of your patients is an elderly lady who is recovering from abdominal surgery. Her Muslim teenage son angrily confronts you on the ward, as he has just found out that his mother has been receiving enoxaparin (low molecular weight heparin) post-operatively. He has learnt through internet research that it is derived from porcine mucosa, and breaches his religious beliefs.

Rank in order the following actions in response to this situation (1 = Most appropriate; 5 = Least appropriate).

A Use a heparin replacement drug which is not of porcine origin and slightly less effective.

B Continue the enoxaparin.

C Cross off the enoxaparin from your patient's chart.

D Interview the patient about her beliefs and whether she would like enoxaparin treatment, given its porcine origin.

E Explore the son's beliefs about enoxaparin and why it shouldn't be given, as well as exceptions to the rules.

Question 101

You are an FY1 covering the night on-call. You are called to see a patient who has been receiving IV fluids and antibiotics for pneumonia. His cannula has stopped working and you have now had two unsuccessful attempts at inserting another one into his arm. The patient refuses to have a cannula sited in his leg.

Rank in order the following actions in response to this situation (1 = Most appropriate; 5 = Least appropriate).

A Call the SHO for help.

B Switch the patient to oral antibiotics.

C Call the anaesthetist as you are having trouble establishing IV access.

D Wait for the patient's regular team to return in the morning to decide how to proceed.

E Attempt to insert a cannula into the patient's leg.

Question 102

You are an FY1 in surgery, with two final-year students attached to your firm. One of the students presents you with an essay that the consultant had asked him to write, before he elects to submit it to the consultant. On checking his work, you realise that large parts of the text have been lifted from an article on the internet.

Choose the THREE most appropriate actions to take in this situation.

A Ask the student to rewrite the essay, and offer to review it again.

B Do not act on your discovery, the document may not yet be referenced correctly.

C Inform the consultant of your findings.

D Speak to the consultant in private and ask his advice about his stance on plagiarism.

E Speak to the student and ask him to explain your findings.

F Read and act on the medical school guidelines for plagiarism.

G Inform the medical school that the student is guilty of plagiarism.

H Talk to the student about integrity and professional conduct as a doctor.

Question 103

You are an FY1 on a medical firm. You have finished your shift and go to the staffroom to retrieve your belongings. You find that your handbag, which had copies of your patient list, has been stolen.

Rank in order the following actions in response to this situation (1 = Most appropriate; 5 = Least appropriate).

A Call the police.

B Inform a senior about your handbag and the documents with patient information.

C Ask the ward staff if they have seen your bag.

D Inform a senior about your handbag and tell them that there was nothing valuable inside.

E Do nothing; it was your own fault for leaving your bag in the staffroom and there was nothing of significant monetary value inside.

Question 104

You are an FY1 on a urology firm. During pre-assessment clinic, one of your patients is found to have a urinary tract infection (UTI) and is sent home with a course of antibiotics. A few days later, you notice that the urine culture results have returned, showing that the infection is resistant to the antibiotic you had prescribed. You have difficulty getting in touch with the GP to inform them of the results.

Rank in order the following actions in response to this situation (1 = Most appropriate; 5 = Least appropriate).

A Call the patient directly and ask him to make an appointment with the GP.

B Call the patient and ask him to see you on the ward for a hospital pharmacy prescription.

C Call the patient and tell him to present to casualty and explain to them the situation.

D Send a letter to the GP, detailing what has happened and what they need to do.

E Cancel the patient's surgery, due to their untreated UTI.

Question 105

You are an FY1 on a paediatrics firm. One of your patients has cerebral palsy and your registrar has objected to physiotherapy, stating that it will not be of benefit. You are unclear of the reason behind this decision. Once the registrar has left the ward, the patient's family insist that you organise intensive physiotherapy for the patient.

Choose the THREE most appropriate actions to take in this situation.

A Sensitively explain to the parents that physiotherapy will not help their child.

B Ask your registrar to speak to the patient and their family.

C Ask the sister on the ward to speak to the parents.
D Speak to the consultant about the management plan.
E Discuss other management options with the registrar.
F Contact the physiotherapists to assess the patient.
G Approach the registrar to better understand the reasons for his decision.
H Recommend to the parents that if they want physiotherapy they will have to pay for it privately.

Question 106

You are on the train on your way back home on Friday night. Your registrar is covering the weekend and calls to ask you to go through the sick patients on your list. You are surrounded by other commuters and have your patient list out in front of you.

Rank in order the following actions in response to this situation (1 = Most appropriate; 5 = Least appropriate).

A Put the list away and discuss the patients from memory.
B Ask the registrar to wait until you are back at home alone, where you will call him back and freely discuss the patients.
C Cover the list such that other commuters cannot read it and discuss the patients with the registrar using initials and not specifying any names.
D Put the list away and inform the registrar that he must identify the patients and you will only be able to answer yes and no to preserve patient confidentiality.
E Tell the registrar that you are on the train and unable to discuss any patients.

Question 107

You are on a surgical firm. Your SHO constantly gives you jobs that she should be doing so that she can spend more time in theatre or leave on time.

Rank in order the following actions in response to this situation (1 = Most appropriate; 5 = Least appropriate).

A Approach your FY1 colleagues and ask for their assistance in completing your additional tasks.
B Confront your SHO and inform her that she is neglecting her duty of care by handing her tasks to you.
C Inform the registrar on the firm that the SHO is neglecting her duties.
D Inform the SHO that her actions are not conducive to the team working cohesively.
E Do not perform the SHO's tasks while she is in theatre.

Question 108

Your registrar, when reviewing an elderly patient, determines that he is fit for discharge and should go home later that afternoon. When you return to complete the patient's discharge paperwork, he seems extremely reluctant.

He goes on to hand you some money to delay his discharge until tomorrow. You are aware that your registrar will be off-site for the rest of the week.

Choose the THREE most appropriate actions to take in this situation.

A Ask for an assessment by physiotherapy to assess his mobility.

B Complete his discharge summary late in the day, so that his drugs do not arrive on time for him to be discharged the same day.

C Reassess the patient and discharge if safe.

D Request that the patient leaves the money in an envelope for you to pick up later.

E Explain that you cannot accept the money but agree to delay his discharge until he feels ready to go home.

F Explore the patient's concerns and reasons for his reluctance to be discharged.

G Ask that the multidisciplinary team reassesses the patient once more prior to discharge and tell the patient to donate the money to charity, since you cannot accept bribes.

H Raise the patient's case at the multidisciplinary meeting, and delay discharge if any concerns arise from the team.

Question 109

You are an FY1 on a busy medical ward. One of your patients has oesophageal cancer with widespread metastases. He is being managed palliatively and is on high doses of morphine which require monitoring. The family request to take the patient home so that he can die in comfort.

Rank in order the following actions in response to this situation (1 = Most appropriate; 5 = Least appropriate).

A Explore whether the family realise the responsibility of taking care of the patient at home.

B Refuse the family's request as he is on medication that requires regular monitoring.

C Ask a senior for advice.

D Establish what the patient's wishes are.

E Contact the palliative care team to ask about support at home.

Question 110

Your FY1 colleague takes you to one side to tell you that her consultant is making inappropriate advances towards her. She feels uncomfortable and does not know who to talk to, as the rest of her team are also male. She reports finding it difficult to do her work and maintain a professional relationship with her team.

Rank in order the following actions in response to this situation (1 = Most appropriate; 5 = Least appropriate).

A Approach the consultant yourself and warn him against pursuing a relationship with your colleague.

B Report the consultant to the GMC.

C Tell your colleague to speak to her consultant and explain that she is feeling uncomfortable.

D Report the consultant to the police for sexual harassment.

E Speak to your registrar for advice.

Question 111

You are an FY1 on a medical rotation. One of your patients is reviewed by the surgical team and a management plan is put in place by the consultant. Your medical registrar disagrees with the plan and tells you not to follow their recommendations.

Rank in order the following actions in response to this situation (1 = Most appropriate; 5 = Least appropriate).

A Action the consultant surgeon's management plan anyway.

B Discuss the management plan with your own consultant.

C Speak to the registrar to understand why he does not agree.

D Ask the surgical team to re-review the patient.

E Approach the surgical team to understand their recommendations.

Question 112

One of the other FY1s you work with has committed a number of errors since they started working. He has managed to pass the first placement, as his consultant is frequently away and unaware of his failings. Since then he has continued to make mistakes, and has developed a reputation for mishaps among the other FY1s. He is now working on the same ward as you and has just missed that a patient's haemoglobin is sufficiently low to warrant a blood transfusion.

Choose the THREE most appropriate actions to take in this situation.

A Talk to your consultant about the errors you have witnessed.

B Approach your colleague's registrar about your colleague's errors.

C Highlight the need for a blood transfusion to your colleague.

D Fill out an incident form about this near miss.

E Order a blood transfusion, correcting the error.

F Report your concerns to the GMC.

G Keep a closer eye on your colleague, correcting his errors, minimising harm to patients.

H Ask the other FY1s about their experiences of his errors.

Question 113

You log into a social network site, while on a lunch break in the doctors' mess. You have just been sent a friend request from a patient you were speaking to this morning and found to have a lot in common with.

Rank in order the following actions in response to this situation (1 = Most appropriate; 5 = Least appropriate).

A Accept the friend request.
B Accept the friend request after reviewing your privacy settings to ensure that she is not exposed to any sensitive information.
C Speak to the patient and explain that you cannot accept the friend request.
D Reject the friend request.
E Deactivate your account and stop using the social networking site.

Question 114

You are covering a busy weekend on-call, where you are bleeped regarding several very unwell patients. You try contacting the on-call SHO, but are unable to reach them. You find your SHO later in the day in the mess. When you explain that you have been trying to contact him, he states that his bleep has been 'playing up' and denies receiving any bleeps.

Rank in order the following actions in response to this situation (1 = Most appropriate; 5 = Least appropriate).

A Contact the on-call registrar when you are next called to a sick patient and require assistance.
B Discuss what has happened with the on-call registrar.
C Complete an incident form.
D Speak to your consultant.
E Tell the other FY1s that the on-call SHO was lazy and useless.

Question 115

You are an FY1 on a renal firm. You receive a bleep from an external line via switchboard. A GP calls expecting to speak to the registrar for advice regarding a patient in her clinic. Your registrar is on annual leave and the consultant is at another hospital seeing private patients.

Rank in order the following actions in response to this situation (1 = Most appropriate; 5 = Least appropriate).

A Tell the GP to go through switchboard and ask to be put through to your renal consultant's mobile.
B Answer the query to the best of your ability.
C Ask the GP to ring the switchboard again and ask to speak to the renal registrar from a sister firm.
D Offer to put the GP in touch with your FY2.
E Tell the GP to speak to the medical registrar or renal registrar on-call.

Question 116

You are an FY1 on a paediatrics firm. You examine a young boy as part of your routine clerking and see some innocuous-looking bruises on his leg which look as though they may have been sustained from a fall while playing. When you are alone with him, he confides in you that they are the result of his parents hitting him at home.

Choose the THREE most appropriate actions to take in this situation.

A Ask the patient if he is aware of the serious nature of his allegations.

B Contact the patient's parents and have a discussion about what has just been said.

C Contact the registrar on-call.

D Document the history and examination findings.

E Ask one of the nurses on the ward to be present in the consultation.

F Ask the patient if he is telling the truth.

G Review previous admissions to casualty to compile a dossier of evidence against the parents.

H Ask the GP whether he has noticed anything untoward about the parents' conduct towards their child.

Question 117

You are an FY1 on an orthopaedic firm. You attend the weekly x-ray meeting with the rest of your surgical team, where the lumbar x-ray of one of your patients is discussed. The radiologist is known to be strict and does not like juniors interrupting him. He suggests an MRI to further characterise an area of abnormality on the scan. You remember the patient stating that she has had a significant amount of metal work in her hip due to her rheumatoid arthritis.

Rank in order the following actions in response to this situation (1 = Most appropriate; 5 = Least appropriate).

A Tell the radiologist about the metal work at the x-ray meeting.

B Tell your consultant of the potential obstacle to an MRI scan, after the meeting.

C Do not say anything, as you are sure the radiologist is aware of the patient's previous surgery.

D Go back to the notes to doublecheck that you are correct about the previous surgery.

E Whisper your concerns to the registrar during the meeting so that she can inform the radiologist of the metal implants.

Question 118

One of your FY1 colleagues reveals that he has completed the assessments for his e-Portfolio by asking senior colleagues who happen to be his friends to certify his competence. You have doubts as to whether the FY1 actually performed the skills being assessed. In contrast, you have been experiencing difficulty in obtaining the same sign-offs.

Choose the THREE most appropriate actions to take in this situation.

A Ask your colleague whether he is competent in the tasks that he has been signed off for.

B Do nothing, as there is no evidence of wrong-doing.

C Inform the GMC of the improper conduct of your colleague and his seniors.

D Speak to your colleague's consultant about your suspicions.

E Inform your consultant that your colleague is being inappropriately signed off.

F Phone your medical defence organisation for anonymous advice.

G Speak to the doctors signing your colleague off and inform them that it is wrong to sign FY1s off without a proper assessment.

H Ask your colleague's seniors to sign you off and check whether or not they assess you, before confirming your competence.

Question 119

Your team is submitting a case report for presentation at an international conference. You send your registrar the poster he had asked you to design, including some content and information which he provided. When it is reviewed and emailed back, you notice that two additional names have been added to the list of authors. You are aware that there is only a short time before the poster must be submitted.

Rank in order the following actions in response to this situation (1 = Most appropriate; 5 = Least appropriate).

A Raise the issue with your consultant, who is also named on the poster.

B Email the two new authors asking about their contribution.

C Include the new names on the poster.

D Remove the new names from the poster.

E Talk to the registrar about the two additional names.

Question 120

You are an FY1 on a medical firm. Your registrar offers you the opportunity to perform your first lumbar puncture on a patient, having practised it on a model. You are both at the patient's bedside, and your registrar has just left to pick up an additional piece of equipment. The patient turns round to ask if you have ever performed the procedure before. You are keen not to make the patient any more anxious than they already are, and want to avoid her from changing her mind about letting you perform the procedure.

Choose the THREE most appropriate actions to take in this situation.

A Inform the patient that you are familiar with the procedure and know how it is performed, and that it is her choice who does it.

B Tell the patient that you have performed the procedure in the past.

C Mention that this is the first lumbar puncture that you are performing.

D Reassure the patient that the registrar will be watching and helping while you perform the procedure.

E Ask the patient whether she will permit the registrar to perform the lumbar puncture.

F Ask the patient whether she would permit you to perform the procedure under close supervision.

G Tell the patient that you haven't, but that she doesn't have a choice as to who does the lumbar puncture.

H Tell the patient that you haven't done it on a person, but you have practised on models and will be closely supervised if she lets you do it, but she does have the choice to opt for the registrar.

Question 121

You are an FY1 on a medical firm. A 23-year-old man who is anxious about discharge on your ward has complained again of retrosternal chest pain. This is the fifth time in the last two weeks that he has described the same complaint. On each occasion, he was fully investigated and the results were always normal.

Rank in order the following actions in response to this situation (1 = Most appropriate; 5 = Least appropriate).

A Do not investigate his chest pain on this occasion.

B Call your registrar and discuss the complaint.

C Provide adequate simple analgesia.

D Examine the patient and start investigations including troponin.

E Write in the notes that the pain is unchanged and the patient is for conservative management only.

Question 122

You are an FY1 on a medical firm. One of your patients is recovering from a stroke and you have been asked to find out about his wishes regarding rehabilitation in a few weeks, and whether he consents to continuing healthcare. The patient communicates with a language board, which you are unfamiliar with and don't know how to use. You recognise that eliciting his wishes is going to be time-consuming and you have a list of other important jobs you must attend to before a consultant ward round in the afternoon.

Rank in order the following actions in response to this situation (1 = Most appropriate; 5 = Least appropriate).

A Take the time to talk to the patient first before completing the important jobs.

B Talk to the patient later when his next of kin arrives to act as an intermediary to relay the patient's responses in order to save time.

C Act in the best interests of the patient and organise transfer to a specialist rehabilitation centre.

D Call the patient's next of kin to find out what their wishes are.

E Ask an experienced nurse to talk to the patient on your behalf.

Question 123

You are returning home after a busy shift. As you wait at the bus stop outside the hospital grounds, you see a passer-by collapse to the ground. Her friend is visibly distressed and calls out for help. You have an early start tomorrow, and you can see your bus arriving in the distance.

Choose the THREE most appropriate actions to take in this situation.

A Catch the bus and leave the casualty alone.
B Start CPR on the casualty.
C Attend to the casualty.
D Assess the patient for signs of life, then catch the bus if she is stable.
E Give advice to the friend of the casualty before catching the bus.
F Stay with the casualty and friend until further help arrives.
G Help carry the casualty to the A&E department of the hospital.
H Call an ambulance.

Question 124

The third-year medical student who is attached to your firm reaches the end of his rotation and brings in his skills logbook. There is a specific section for FY1 shadowing which he asks you to sign. He has only attended ward rounds twice during his three-month placement and has not stayed with you long enough to learn what you do during your day.

Rank in order the following actions in response to this situation (1 = Most appropriate; 5 = Least appropriate).

A Sign the student off – he is only in his third year.
B Inform the medical school that you cannot sign off the student.
C Offer to sign the student off if he spends three days with you and impresses you.
D Explore why the student has been absent and offer advice.
E Refuse to sign the student off.

Question 125

Your FY1 colleague prepares the equipment to take urgent bloods from one of the patients on the gastroenterology ward. She learns that the patient has hepatitis B and refuses to bleed him despite your efforts to convince her otherwise, as she does not want to put her own health at risk.

Rank in order the following actions in response to this situation (1 = Most appropriate; 5 = Least appropriate).

A Take the patient's blood sample yourself.
B Tell your colleague sensitively that her decision is irresponsible and that she should not refuse to take the patient's blood.

C Accept your colleague's decision not to take the patient's blood and bleed the patient yourself when necessary.

D Tell your colleague to use two pairs of gloves for safety in future.

E Refuse to take the patient's blood yourself, for your own safety.

Question 126

You are treating a young woman for the injuries she has sustained to her arms. While the A&E clerking notes state that these were due to a fall, on further questioning, you elicit that her husband has been increasingly abusive to her due to an alcohol problem. She maintains that she does not wish for any action to be taken, and wants an opportunity to work on their relationship.

Rank in order the following actions in response to this situation (1 = Most appropriate; 5 = Least appropriate).

A Inform the police, as she has been assaulted.

B Document your findings in the patient's notes, in case the patient wishes to press charges.

C Respect her confidentiality and do not do anything.

D Provide details of domestic violence help lines and advise her on the procedure, should she change her mind and wish to take the matter further.

E Contact her partner and arrange an appointment to see him.

Question 127

A patient who was admitted with severe shortness of breath is found to have pneumocystis pneumonia (PCP), secondary to a previously undiagnosed HIV infection. The patient requests that this information is omitted from his discharge summary, so that his GP does not find out.

Rank in order the following actions in response to this situation (1 = Most appropriate; 5 = Least appropriate).

A Include the diagnosis of HIV in the discharge summary, regardless of whether the patient agrees or not, as the information must be recorded.

B Agree to omit the diagnosis from the discharge summary, but then inform the GP practice anyway as the GP has a right to know.

C Respect the wishes of the patient and do not include the diagnosis in the discharge summary.

D Explain the importance of recording the diagnosis in the discharge summary and the potential risk he poses. If he continues to object, respect his wishes and do not include this information in the letter to the GP.

E Explain to the patient that he poses a risk to the staff at the GP practice and they have a right to know. If he continues to object, state that you must break confidentiality to act in the best interests of your colleagues in the GP surgery.

Question 128

You are an FY1 doing a taster week in anaesthetics. You are keen to impress the consultant and have researched the various techniques used for airway management. On the morning of a theatre list, the consultant has difficultly intubating one of the patients. The nurses recognise that there is a problem and bring in the emergency tracheostomy set and contact the Intensive Therapy Unit (ITU). The consultant ignores their concerns and continues to try to intubate. You notice that the patient is going blue and her oxygen saturations have been falling for the last five minutes, and attempts to ventilate the patient with bag and mask have failed.

Rank in order the following actions in response to this situation (1 = Most appropriate; 5 = Least appropriate).

A Prepare the tracheostomy set.

B Inform the anaesthetist that the patient is turning blue.

C Do not disturb the anaesthetist and allow him to concentrate on intubating the patient.

D Ask the anaesthetist if you can attempt intubation with a fresh pair of hands.

E Intervene by suggesting to the consultant that intubation should be abandoned and the patient requires an emergency tracheostomy.

Question 129

You are an FY1 working on a specialist stroke ward. Currently there are also two medical outliers on your ward, and a consultant from another ward will come to see these patients with the junior members of his team. This morning, the visiting consultant comes to review his patients but then asks you to complete the jobs, since his own juniors are busy on another ward. When informed of this, your own consultant berates you in front of your entire team, stating that your priority should be your own patients.

Choose the THREE most appropriate actions to take in this situation.

A Ask your consultant what he would like you to do about the jobs you have already accepted.

B Refuse to complete jobs in future for the other medical team.

C Call the visiting consultant's juniors and hand back the jobs.

D Comply with the visiting consultant's requests for the day, if they do not compromise the care that you provide.

E Inform the visiting consultant that you will not be able to regularly complete jobs for his team.

F Only complete the visiting consultant's requests after you have completed tasks for your own patients.

G Privately speak to your consultant explaining that patient care has not been compromised by accepting the additional workload.

H Complete only the urgent jobs for the other medical team, leaving the remaining non-urgent jobs to be handed back the next morning.

Question 130

You are an FY1 on a medical firm. One of your FY1 colleagues comes to your ward in the morning. He reports feeling hungover as he went to the mess party last night. He asks you to give him some IV fluids and paracetamol from the treatment room to help him recover in time for the morning ward round.

Choose the THREE most appropriate actions to take in this situation.

A Report your colleague to your senior.

B Offer to cover for him for the next hour so that he can recover.

C Provide your colleague with paracetamol from your own supply.

D Tell your colleague that he should go home if he is not feeling well.

E Suggest that it is unprofessional to come to work in this state.

F Provide your colleague with paracetamol from the ward, and ensure that the ward sister does not see.

G Give your colleague the IV fluids to help him recover quickly.

H Politely explain that you are busy preparing for the ward round and that he should contact the ward sister for help.

Question 131

You are an FY1 in Ear, Nose and Throat (ENT) surgery. One of your patients develops stridor post-operatively and needs an urgent senior review. You call your registrar who refuses to see the patient but offers basic instructions as he is busy in clinic and is not on-call until after 5pm. You know the consultant on-call but are aware that he gets very angry when called by junior doctors. You have already followed the basic advice.

Rank in order the following actions in response to this situation (1 = Most appropriate; 5 = Least appropriate).

A Wait until 5pm to call the registrar again.

B Try calling the registrar again and insist that he reviews the patient.

C Ask the nurses for advice on whom to contact.

D Contact the on-call consultant.

E Attempt to manage the patient yourself.

Question 132

You are doing a placement in general practice. You are informed that a newly registered patient is at the reception requesting a repeat prescription. Your senior is in the middle of a busy clinic, and all the appointment slots have been filled. The patient asks you to take the repeat prescription form to your senior to be signed in between seeing patients.

Rank in order the following actions in response to this situation (1 = Most appropriate; 5 = Least appropriate).

A Ask the patient to go to casualty to pick up an emergency supply of drugs until an appointment can be made.

B Review the drugs on the repeat prescription.

C If there is nothing urgent that needs to be prescribed, ask the patient to make an appointment at the earliest opportunity next week, and do not arrange for him to have any drugs to go home with.

D Contact the patient's previous GP for an accurate drug history.

E If there is nothing urgent that should be prescribed, ask the patient to make an appointment at the earliest opportunity, and arrange for a one-week supply to be issued so that he does not run out in the interim.

Question 133

You are an FY1 on an orthopaedics rotation. A patient has returned to your ward following a hip replacement. The nurses inform you that she is in distress and asks you to go to see her, as she is attempting to pull out her cannula. Her partner is waiting outside the ward, as it is not yet visiting hours.

Choose the THREE most appropriate actions to take in this situation.

A Assist in removing the patient's cannula to calm her down.

B Ask the ward sister to call the husband in to see her.

C Explore the reasons why the patient may be distressed and examine her.

D Inform one of your senior colleagues of the situation.

E Give the patient a sedative to calm her down.

F Give the patient analgesia.

G Ask the nursing staff to help calm her down.

H Do nothing, as this is likely a transient response which she will recover from.

Question 134

You are an FY1 on a medical firm and your consultant is giving a grand round presentation. Two of your FY1 colleagues are talking to each other two rows behind you, disturbing you and those around them.

Rank in order the following actions in response to this situation (1 = Most appropriate; 5 = Least appropriate).

A Put your hand up and inform the presenter that you cannot hear him, because of background noise.

B Ignore the issue and do nothing.

C Tell your FY1 colleagues directly to stop talking, at the risk of distracting others.

D Ignore the issue, but approach your colleagues after the lecture to inform them of the noise that they made.

E Ask the person behind you to pass on the message to your FY1 colleagues that they are being disruptive.

Question 135

You are an FY1 on a colorectal firm. You are in a busy pre-assessment clinic, for patients who are due to undergo elective surgery next week. You cannot find the notes for the next patient, who is due to undergo a hernia repair. He has already been waiting three hours to see you and starts shouting in the waiting area, calling you an incompetent doctor.

Choose the THREE most appropriate actions to take in this situation.

A Ask someone senior to come and help you deal with the patient.
B Leave the patient to wait until the notes are found.
C See the patient without access to his notes.
D Ask a nurse to look for the notes while you see the patient.
E Ask him why he is shouting.
F Apologise to the patient for the delay.
G Inform him that you will not see him if he continues to shout.
H Inform him that it is unacceptable for him to shout at you.

Question 136

You are an FY1 on a medical firm and covering for one of your colleagues who is on annual leave. One of the patients you are covering has had recent CT scans to investigate the cause of her protracted vomiting. You review the report with your consultant, which states that the findings are likely brain metastases from a previously diagnosed breast cancer. The consultant is late for a clinic and tells you to break the bad news to the patient. Since you do not know the patient case very well, you do not feel comfortable doing this.

Rank in order the following actions in response to this situation (1 = Most appropriate; 5 = Least appropriate).

A Tell the patient the findings.
B Get the information you need from the nurse and explain what is happening.
C Tell the consultant that you are not comfortable doing this.
D Get the information you need from the notes and explain the findings to the patient.
E Explain to the patient that your consultant will return in the afternoon to explain the results.

Question 137

Being slightly late, you rush into the weekly teaching sessions that are held for foundation trainees following a busy morning. The sessions are designed to be 'bleep-free' and the administration staff, who collect bleeps at the start, only interrupt the sessions to call you if there is an emergency. You have forgotten to hand in your bleep and it has just gone off during the session.

Rank in order the following actions in response to this situation (1 = Most appropriate; 5 = Least appropriate).

A Answer the bleep and do the jobs you are asked to do.

B Leave the teaching session to hand the bleep to the administration staff, informing them that it has just gone off.

C Ignore the bleep and take the battery out so that it does not cause further interruptions.

D Ignore the bleep on this occasion but answer it if they continue to attempt to contact you.

E Answer the bleep and ask that they contact your SHO to complete any jobs, as you are in teaching.

Question 138

You are an FY1 on a medical firm. Your consultant asks you to make an alteration to a patient's notes from an entry made on a consultant ward round last week, which had stated that the patient was medically fit for discharge. The patient was subsequently found to have a low haemoglobin level that required an emergency blood transfusion.

Rank in order the following actions in response to this situation (1 = Most appropriate; 5 = Least appropriate).

A Make the change requested by the consultant.

B Report the matter to the clinical director.

C Inform the patient of the mistake and your consultant's request.

D Make a note of the conversation between you and the consultant.

E Inform the GMC.

Question 139

You are an FY1 on an evening ward cover on-call shift. You have 30 minutes remaining before the handover meeting and you review your remaining jobs. You are deciding which order to do outstanding jobs and are wary of handing over anything trivial to the night team as you were grilled by the registrar last time you did this.

Rank in order the following actions in response to this situation (1 = Most appropriate; 5 = Least appropriate).

A Review the elderly patient who fell out of their bed about an hour ago, but is clinically well.

B Cannulate a patient who is due to have IV antibiotics in the next two hours for community-acquired pneumonia.

C Review the patient you have just been bleeped about, who is complaining again of right iliac fossa pain and is being treated for query appendicitis.

D Recheck the potassium level on a computer for a patient that you bled at the start of the evening shift following an earlier blood test demonstrating a high potassium level, for which no treatment was started.

E Speak to the concerned family of a patient who is not normally under your care.

Question 140

You are an FY1 on a surgical rotation. At the start of the firm you review the on-call rota and find that you will be working significantly more on-call shifts than any of the other surgical FY1s, even though the number that you are scheduled to do is compliant with your employment contract.

Rank in order the following actions in response to this situation (1 = Most appropriate; 5 = Least appropriate).

A Speak to medical staffing in confidence to discuss the rota.

B Refuse to attend the excess shifts for which you have been scheduled.

C Ignore the issue; the rota is compliant with your contract, and you do not have grounds to complain.

D Ask your fellow FY1s to accept some of your shifts so that the balance is fairer.

E Highlight the issue to your consultant.

Question 141

You are an FY1 on a colorectal firm. A patient who is three days post-operative is visibly dyspnoeic and distressed, requiring 40 per cent oxygen to saturate above 90. Following your surgical registrar's instruction, you have called the medical registrar on-call who is refusing to see the patient due to a very busy take.

Rank in order the following actions in response to this situation (1 = Most appropriate; 5 = Least appropriate).

A Call the respiratory registrar for a review.

B Ask the medical registrar for advice as opposed to a review.

C Start the patient on antibiotics.

D Order an urgent chest x-ray.

E Examine the patient.

Question 142

You are an FY1 on a medical firm. You have a patient with gangrenous toes that require debridement or amputation, and your consultant has asked a vascular consultant to assume responsibility for care. The vascular consultant comes to review the patient and arranges surgical intervention but appears reluctant to take over the patient's care insisting that the patient is best cared for under the medical team. When asked by your own consultant, the vascular consultant states that the patient refused transfer to another ward as justification for not taking over care. You believe that he is being dishonest as this was not the same reason the vascular consultant gave you.

Rank in order the following actions in response to this situation (1 = Most appropriate; 5 = Least appropriate).

A Confirm with the patient that she does not wish to move wards.

B Speak to the vascular consultant again to confirm his story.

C Express your concerns to your consultant.

D Ask advice from the vascular team about the patient's care.

E Do not act on your suspicions.

Question 143

You are covering a busy weekend ward cover on-call shift. You arrive onto one of the medical wards, where the ward sister berates you for taking so long to arrive and threatens you with a formal complaint. You were attending to a sick patient on another ward, and you are not aware of any urgent jobs on the ward you have just arrived onto.

Rank in order the following actions in response to this situation (1 = Most appropriate; 5 = Least appropriate).

A Explore why the sister is angry at you for arriving late to non-urgent jobs.

B Refuse to complete any jobs until the sister is polite to you.

C Inform the sister that you were busy on another ward.

D Tell the sister to complain, as you can defend your actions.

E Threaten to complain about the sister's behaviour.

Question 144

You are an FY1 on a medical firm. Your shift ended 15 minutes ago and you are heading out of the hospital. Just as you are walking out of the door of the doctor's office, your bleep goes off.

Rank in order the following actions in response to this situation (1 = Most appropriate; 5 = Least appropriate).

A Ignore the bleep as your shift has ended and you have already handed over.

B Answer the bleep and take down the details of the job. If it is not too demanding, do the job.

C Answer the bleep and take down the details of the job, so that you can hand it over to the on-call team.

D Answer the bleep and assess the call. Tell the caller to contact the on-call team if it is a matter that does not specifically require your input.

E Answer the bleep and do the job regardless of the nature of the task, as you are still on-site.

Question 145

You are an FY1 on a medical firm. You find out that the two medical students attached to your team had access to the questions that came up in a recent examination one week before it was set by the medical school. The results of the test contribute to the overall academic ranking at the end of the year, which influences the scores for foundation training.

Rank in order the following actions in response to this situation (1 = Most appropriate; 5 = Least appropriate).

A Inform your SHO of the issue.
B Report the issue to the medical school and name the students involved.
C Report the issue to the medical school without naming the students involved, so that the problem can be investigated.
D Report the issue to the undergraduate education department at your hospital.
E Make it clear that what the students did was unacceptable and warn them not to do it again.

Question 146

You are an FY1 completing a surgical night on-call. The locum SHO who is responsible for accepting A&E referrals has not turned up for the night and the consultant who is on-call has informed you that you will assume this role. There are several patients who have been referred to you by the A&E doctors. There is pressure on you to discharge two of them after your surgical review. The registrar will be busy assisting in theatre.

Rank in order the following actions in response to this situation (1 = Most appropriate; 5 = Least appropriate).

A Assess the referrals case by case, refusing the referrals as you judge appropriate.
B Discharge the patients who have been earmarked by A&E as appropriate for discharge, after reviewing them.
C Assess the referrals individually and accept them all.
D Bleep the registrar after reviewing but before accepting each individual patient.
E Call the orthopaedic registrar or SHO who are less busy, when you need advice.

Question 147

You are an FY1 on a surgical firm. You are in a pre-assessment clinic while your seniors are all in theatre. Your next patient is a practising doctor. He admits to drinking excessive amounts of alcohol, stating that work has been very demanding lately. He is concerned that he will lose his job and asks you not to tell anyone of his drinking habits.

Rank in order the following actions in response to this situation (1 = Most appropriate; 5 = Least appropriate).

A Determine the extent of his drinking problem. If there is no immediate danger to patient safety, offer him information on support groups and suggest he takes some time off work.
B Contact his employers to determine whether there have been any issues surrounding patient safety at work.
C Report the matter to the GMC.

D Request that he comes back to see you or his GP if the problem worsens or if he feels he is endangering patients.

E Speak to a senior colleague for advice on how the situation should be managed.

Question 148

You are an FY1 on a surgical firm. You and your SHO have completed all the jobs you are required to do, three hours before the end of your shift. Your SHO has a friend's party to attend this evening and wishes to leave early.

Choose the THREE most appropriate actions to take in this situation.

A Explain that she should remain until the end of the shift in case any emergencies arise.

B Ask that she redirects the bleep to the on-call doctor for that evening.

C Review all the jobs to ensure that there is nothing outstanding and that you are aware of the sickest patients.

D Allow her to leave and take her bleep, calling the registrar if anything beyond your competence arises.

E Insist that she stays to complete her shift.

F Ask that she clears this with your registrar.

G Let her leave as you should be able to handle everything yourself until the end of the shift.

H Tell your consultant that your SHO has left early to attend a personal engagement.

Question 149

You are an FY1 on a surgical firm. One of your patients has an unexplained rise in creatinine that requires further investigation and your consultant requests that you get a review by the renal team. The renal registrar calls you in the afternoon and berates you for making an inappropriate referral and wasting her time.

Rank in order the following actions in response to this situation (1 = Most appropriate; 5 = Least appropriate).

A Apologise before clarifying the advice from the registrar.

B Apologise to the renal registrar for the referral and explain that you were instructed to make it.

C Ask the registrar why the referral was inappropriate, to prevent you repeating this mistake.

D Explain to the registrar that you have already conducted the basic investigations before her call and update her with the results before asking her input.

E Tell the registrar that her threatening behaviour is not warranted.

Question 150

You are an FY1 covering a night on-call. During a quiet morning with no jobs, you are approached by a housekeeper working on the ward, who asks if you would mind taking a blood sample from her to send to the labs. She explains that it is a fasting sample for a lipid profile ordered by her GP, and that she is diabetic and keen to eat. Her GP is on the hospital system and she would otherwise have to wait until 9am to visit the phlebotomy service downstairs, where she would join the long queue.

Rank in order the following actions in response to this situation (1 = Most appropriate; 5 = Least appropriate).

A Gather equipment from the phlebotomy department and come back to bleed the housekeeper.

B Take a blood sample from the housekeeper on the ward and send it to the labs.

C Sensitively refuse to bleed the housekeeper, as you will not be able to check the results later.

D Decline the request to bleed her as your patients must take priority.

E Ask the ward sister if she minds you bleeding the housekeeper on the ward.

6: Practice Answers

Question 1

D, B, A, E, C

Probity is an important aspect of practice. In a situation such as this, one must avoid lying to the patient. With this in mind, there is no concrete diagnosis of cancer and further tests would be appropriate before the diagnosis is established. Best practice would involve a senior colleague breaking any bad news to the patient, although this is not always practical.

Option D: This would be the most appropriate course of action, as you are requesting that a senior colleague discuss the findings with the patient, while remaining honest.

Option B: This is the next best option, as you are awaiting further information before discussing the findings with the patient. However, as a senior colleague is not present, this is less appropriate than Option D.

Option A: This allows for a sensitive private discussion with the patient, exploring his fears and concerns. However, handing your bleep inconveniences a colleague and potentially compromises the care of other patients. Without the full results available, the scope of the consultation is limited and thus not ideal.

Option E: This is not as appropriate as the above options, given the absence of definitive results and of a close relative or senior colleague.

Option C: This is the least appropriate response as you are giving the patient false hope and imparting incorrect information.

Question 2

A, E, B, D, C

The most concerning aspect of this scenario is the threat to patient care and safety. One must evaluate the potential risk to patients in permitting the nurse to continue working. The issue requires sensitive handling to determine the exact nature of events and to protect a professional relationship. It is worth noting that a minor criminal offence has been committed in the act of stealing prescription medication.

Option A: This is the most appropriate response as it allows you to establish the facts of the event witnessed. If the nurse is indeed self-medicating, this places patients at risk and it is your responsibility to prevent her from working.

Option E: By informing the ward sister, you are acting promptly in the interests of patients. This action does not, however, allow the nurse to explain herself, and may result in the incident being handled insensitively.

Option B: This response is not as appropriate as the options above. Discussing the matter with your consultant would take steps towards resolving the issue and preventing the nurse from working that day, however, there would be a substantial delay in which patients may be exposed to harm.

Option D: This is not an appropriate response and would be excessive since facts have yet to be established about what you have observed. Furthermore, protocol favours resolution of issues at a local level before escalating the matter to senior authorities.

Option C: This is the least appropriate response as you have potentially placed patients at risk by omission.

Question 3

D, F, H

In a scenario such as this it is easy to get side-tracked by the potential criminal act that may have occurred. However, patient welfare must be your top priority and, as such, you must ensure that their condition has not acutely deteriorated, leading to these claims. This must not, however, be used as an excuse to ignore the patient's allegations, and their concerns must be acknowledged.

Option D: This validates the patient's concerns and ensures that they are investigated. This approach deals with the situation sensitively as you make enquiries with the nurses looking after the patient, without making any accusations.

Option F: This allows for further details of the incident to be established and demonstrates to the patient that his concerns are being acknowledged.

Option H: This option is the most appropriate response, given the patient's medical history. The alleged incident may be a symptom of acute delirium or worsening dementia. It would therefore be necessary to fully examine the patient to ensure that medical treatment is not required. Regardless of the outcome, the claims should still be investigated.

Option A: Completing an incident form is appropriate. However, this is less of a priority as it does not deal with the situation at hand. Such measures can be undertaken once more important actions have been performed.

Option B: You must not discriminate against a patient on the basis of their medical condition. Therefore you must not reassure the patient without establishing the facts.

Option C: This is wholly inappropriate and may constitute an assault on the patient.

Option E: This response may help to ascertain the baseline cognitive state of the patient and discuss experiences with the rest of the healthcare team.

However, this is less appropriate than other options that are available which deal with the situation with greater urgency.

Option G: This is an excessive response in the absence of evidence of any criminal act.

Question 4

B, C, F

Working as part of a team involves dependence upon others to fulfil their roles and responsibilities. In this question, the tardiness of your colleague is likely to have an impact on an already busy surgical firm, and indirectly, on the care of your patients. The situation requires a careful approach towards your colleague, who may be in need of support due to external pressure. You must also consider your own well-being and the practicality of undertaking a demanding job by yourself. Many of the responses in this question are inappropriate, requiring comparison against each other.

Option B: This is an appropriate response. By speaking to your colleague, you are addressing the issue at hand. Making her aware of the problem without involving an additional party is in the interest of maintaining a healthy professional relationship.

Option C: By working harder to compensate for your colleague's absence, you are attempting to rectify the situation but acknowledge that this is not a long-term solution. While not ideal, this response is more appropriate than the others below.

Option F: Discussing the matter with your seniors also addresses the situation. Senior doctors such as your FY2 may be able to help you in the interim by increasing their presence on the ward and relieving the pressure on you. The registrar may attempt to talk to your colleague to establish if there are underlying issues that need to be addressed.

Option A: This action is inappropriate. Discussion with the nurses may adversely affect both the working relationship between yourself and your colleague, and her relationship with the nurses. This discussion will not bring about any solutions to the current problem.

Option D: Calling your colleague's partner may threaten your professional relationship with her. It may be perceived as a betrayal of trust, especially if her partner is unaware of the reason for her late attendance to work.

Option E: Ignoring the situation and waiting for others to notice does not deal with the situation directly, and is potentially putting patients at risk.

Option G: Similarly to Option A, this response involves additional parties whose involvement will not be conducive to producing a resolution. This action may adversely affect multiple professional relationships.

Option H: Unaware of the circumstances surrounding the recent poor punctuality, it would not be appropriate to suggest that your colleague make up the additional hours. Such an approach may be insensitive and negatively impact upon your working relationship.

Question 5

D, E, F

It is not uncommon for patients to attempt to self-discharge against medical advice. These events can be challenging as the patient must be assessed for capacity to make such a decision. If the patient demonstrates a lack of capacity, you must act in his or her best interests. This may involve holding them against their will while they are treated under your care.

Option D: Calming the patient down verbally is the best course of action. An assessment may reveal the cause of the delirium. This would facilitate treatment and may resolve the confusion, after which he will be able to make a valid decision as to whether or not he wishes to stay.

Option E: This response is suitable provided you do not place either yourself, your colleagues or the patient at excessive risk. While this patient does pose a risk, this course of action is necessary in light of the other options. As above, an assessment may aid in the further management of the patient.

Option F: Calling security to assist in restraining an abusive patient is an appropriate response. This patient needs treatment and is highly unlikely to have insight into his actions. With assistance from security, it may be possible to assess the patient and establish whether or not he has capacity, at which point treatment can commence as necessary.

Option A: Moving the patient to a locked ward may have a place in further management, but should not be considered in the immediate setting as he currently requires active medical intervention.

Option B: This is an inappropriate response, since the patient is acutely confused and has no clear evidence of psychiatric illness.

Option C: Sedation may have a role in patients that pose a serious risk to themselves or others. However, it should not be used for the convenience of other patients or staff. It may be used to prevent a patient lacking capacity from leaving, where other methods of restraint have been exhausted or are unsafe to use.

Option G: This is not an appropriate response. The patient lacks capacity and thus you must act in his best interests.

Option H: This is an appropriate response, however, the patient requires immediate attention. This option would present a delay in management and is not as suitable as other answers.

Question 6

E, A, D, B, C

This scenario tests professional integrity. Declining gifts from a grateful patient can be very difficult. It is important to ensure that a gift is proportional to the level of treatment the patient has received. For instance, receiving a box of chocolates at discharge following a period of care is far more reasonable than receiving a watch following a clinical consultation. Judging the appropriateness of a gift can sometimes be challenging, but you must use your initiative and apply your moral values. Accepting gifts on a recurrent basis, as in the question, may have been appropriate in the first instance. However, questions must be raised on subsequent encounters. You must examine whether the patient feels obliged to continue presenting gifts or whether she believes that they are a form of payment. You must always be able to defend your professional integrity and justify your response.

Option E: This is the most appropriate response. Exploring the reasons for the gifts may shed light on why the patient is continually offering them and could enable you to successfully stop such gifts without causing offence and harming the doctor–patient relationship.

Option A: Asking your consultant to intervene on your behalf may have a positive effect. Your consultant is likely to possess experience to approach the topic of gifts sensitively and resolve the matter, while addressing any underlying reasons.

Option D: Accepting the gift on behalf of the healthcare team, while not the most suitable option does make clear that the patient is not directly rewarding you for her treatment and that credit is due to the entire multidisciplinary team.

Option B: Declining the bottle of wine sensitively may signal to the patient that gifts are not required. Accepting it on insistence will limit any offence caused. This response is not ideal as it does not address the issue.

Option C: This is the least appropriate answer. Accepting the gift without question fails to address the underlying issue, and will normalise this custom. This answer fails to explore the views and beliefs of the patient.

Question 7

B, C, E, D, A

Working with colleagues in high-pressure environments can sometimes be quite challenging. While accepting that your colleagues in other professions have many tasks to fulfil, you must make clear the urgency of critical jobs. In this scenario, a patient is critically ill and needs urgent attention. The allocated task has not been performed and it is important to find out why. There may be a good reason for the nurse to withhold the antibiotics, such as an allergy. However, having conveyed the immediacy of the situation to her, she ideally should have contacted you in the instance that she was unable to administer the drug. The priority here remains the patient and, as such, the responses should be ranked in order of safely providing treatment first.

Option B: Speaking to the nurse looking after the patient may reveal important information as to why the drug has not been administered.

Where the drug has not been given, you should endeavour to discover why before administering it yourself. This will prevent you from unknowingly causing harm to the patient.

Option C: Without knowing why the drug hasn't been given, in the interests of patient safety, you should ensure the suitability of your prescription before administering it promptly. While you may not have administered this particular antibiotic before, you should have the skills necessary to set up an IV infusion. Antibiotics are the most suitable medication in this instance and must not be delayed because you cannot find a nurse.

Option E: Discussing the case with a senior will offer a more experienced insight into the next course of action. This discussion is concerned with direct patient management and is therefore preferred to the following responses.

Option D: Filling out the form is a professional responsibility. However, there is no urgency in completing it and tasks involving direct patient care must be attended to first.

Option A: Withholding antibiotics is inappropriate. The patient may still benefit from the antibiotics and the choice to start palliative care should not be taken without senior review and until active management has either failed, or is known to be futile.

Question 8

E, D, H

This question focuses on patient care and probity. You must ensure patient safety above all else, but nevertheless, you must also protect a patient's faith in the profession and your own integrity. Guidance from the GMC is quite clear on the subject of clinical error and patient harm. The immediate concerns should be to put matters right, followed by a prompt apology and explanation to the patient. This question contains multiple appropriate responses, some containing subtle differences from the others. You should approach such scenarios by prioritising what must be done first, followed by actions that are more fitting than others.

Option E: This is an appropriate response. Superseded by removing the cause of harm and treating the patient appropriately, GMC guidance indicates that the patient should be informed promptly. The patient has a right to know and this will help them to retain faith and trust in the profession.

Option D: It is imperative to assess the patient. By doing so, you will be able to ascertain whether or not the patient has come to harm because of the error. Any side-effects of the overdose need to be treated immediately to protect the patient from further harm.

Option H: Correcting the error is important. This is an immediate action undertaken to ensure that the source of harm is removed and further harm does not occur. Leaving this action until later is irresponsible as the patient is still at risk from a continuing overdose. You should always document your actions in the patient's notes, and are at the same time taking measures to inform the patient's usual team.

Option A: This response is partially correct. Rectifying the mistake is important, but notifying the nurse that the matter is resolved is inappropriate and dishonest. Further actions, as outlined above, need to be fulfilled before the matter can be said to be resolved.

Option B: This response is clearly inappropriate. You must rectify the mistake yourself. It is not wise to leave it for someone else to correct as it may be overlooked and thus allow the overdosing to continue.

Option C: This is an appropriate response; however, more pressing action is required before you fill in the incident form. In order of priority, it is more important to inform the patient of the error before completing the incident form.

Option F: Highlighting the error as opposed to correcting it is an important distinction. Notifying the consultant in the morning will mean that the error is picked up and amended, but the safest practice is to correct the error immediately. For instance, the morning ward round may be delayed, and the patient may receive a further double dose before the consultant is able to come around. Furthermore, documenting the error in the notes as per the response above, is better practice than verbally informing the consultant, given that your actions are legally recorded.

Option G: Calling a senior is a good safety net. However, in this instance, you are suitably qualified to resolve this matter yourself and inform the patient. If there are any further issues or you do not feel comfortable with the situation, you should not hesitate to involve a senior.

Question 9

E, C, D, B, A

This is a challenging scenario in which you are faced with a young patient in need of treatment, without her parents being present. There are two main areas being tested in this question: confidentiality and consent. The situation is complicated, with a young person who is intelligent and seemingly able to consent, yet is, at the same time, unwilling to involve her parents or allow you to contact them. You must act in the best interests of the patient and, additionally, respect her rights.

Option E: This is the most appropriate answer. The question indicates that the patient will require a transfusion in the coming hours, thus you have time to explore the patient's concerns. There may be some underlying child protection issues to be uncovered. Furthermore, such a discussion may help to convince the patient to call her parents herself.

Option C: Transfusing the patient is acceptable. She has capacity to consent to the transfusion, which is in her best interests, and you are given no reason to call her parents. GMC guidance in these matters does state that you should encourage her to call her parents nonetheless.

Option D: While it is appropriate to encourage the patient to call her parents, contacting them yourself is inappropriate and breaches this young person's right to confidentiality. If the patient had refused the transfusion, an argument for calling her parents may have existed, as you would need to act in her best interests. This is not the case here.

Option B: This answer is inappropriate. Not only does the patient have capacity, GMC guidance states that you should endeavour to inform the patient if you are going to break confidentiality. There are a few exceptions to this, however, they do not appear in this case.

Option A: This is the least favourable response. Refusing medical treatment when the patient is in need and has consented with capacity is not acceptable. Furthermore, breaking confidentiality is not justifiable. If the treatment is in the child's best interests and the child has capacity, parents of patients cannot refuse the treatment on their behalf.

Question 10

A, B, H

Striking the perfect work/life balance is seldom possible. Balancing work commitments with external responsibilities is challenging, as any task that may have been overlooked must be addressed, particularly if there is potential to compromise patient care. One approach is to hand over jobs to the on-call team. Ideally, work life should not encroach on your personal life, however, it is necessary to possess organisational and coping skills to prevent this. This question is testing your assessment of a situation where multiple factors have to be considered and weighed against the effect on your plans. It is important to note that patient care and effective handover are also considerations in this question.

Option A: This is an appropriate response, despite not being ideal. Calling the FY1 one hour later is not dealing with a matter of patient care immediately. At the same time, the matter is not in need of immediate attention as the insulin is a morning dose.

Option B: This response immediately addresses the issue. By calling the medical registrar, you are ensuring that the job has been handed over with sufficient information. The medical registrar may prescribe the insulin himself, or may in turn ask the FY1 to do so.

Option H: This option is not ideal but it is the third best option available. By calling the ward, you are able to attend to your engagements and have handed over the task. Handing over the job to someone who is not capable of completing the task but who must in turn hand it over, is not best practice but is acceptable.

Option C: Waiting until morning is not an appropriate answer. There is a potential risk to patient care. There is a chance that you may be late on the way to work, in which case the patient may be given the wrong dose of insulin.

Option D: This is not an appropriate answer. If the situation was an emergency, and no one was contactable, there may be scope to return to the hospital yourself. Given the alternative options, this is not a suitable answer.

Option E: This is marginally better than Option D. The risk to patient care exists, in that the longer it takes to resolve this matter, the more likely you are to forget about it. It is still not an appropriate answer for the situation.

Option F: This is an inappropriate answer. There is no guarantee that the FY1 on-call will check her phone, and does not constitute an adequate handover. Furthermore, sending confidential patient information via a text message is in violation of the Data Protection Act.

Option G: This is not an appropriate answer given the other options. Delaying the patient's insulin in the morning is potentially causing harm to the patient, albeit in a mild fashion. There is also the risk that you may arrive late in the morning, leading to someone else prescribing the insulin at the pre-amended dose and causing the patient direct harm.

Question 11

B, E, C, A, D

This scenario focuses on your ability to manage problems that arise when working with others. It is important to maintain good working relationships with your team. However, you must take the necessary steps if patient care is compromised by the absence of senior support. In addition, working beyond your means is not sustainable and may itself impact on the level of care you provide for patients. Any problems that do arise should be dealt with at a local level, before being escalated as necessary.

Option B: This allows for the problem to be addressed directly, while maintaining a good working relationship with your registrar.

Option E: This option escalates the issue to a more senior colleague and deals with the problem at hand. However, it bypasses the registrar and may adversely affect your relationship with him.

Option C: This is not ideal, as it does not aim to resolve the issue. Speaking to a colleague may provide an opportunity to obtain advice, but will not improve the situation. It is, however, more suitable than the remaining options.

Option A: This option may be impractical, as your registrar may be in the middle of an operation, compromising the care of the patient in theatre. In addition, it will negatively impact on your relationship with him. While addressing the issue, it is not ideal to make demands instead of discussing your concerns, and the registrar may not be receptive to improving the situation.

Option D: This is the least suitable option, as it escalates the issue inappropriately and bypasses senior colleagues and your registrar, who are better equipped to resolve the situation.

Question 12

B, D, H

This question is related to balancing patient welfare against respecting the management plans formulated by senior colleagues. You must ensure that the consultant's decision was well informed and took into consideration the reasons behind your concerns. If these were not factored into your consultant's decision, it may be worth reviewing the case to determine whether additional measures are needed before discharge. Ideally, this should be with your consultant who took the initial decision. However, this is not one of the options available and you must therefore weigh up the options which are presented.

Option B: This allows for the case to be reviewed before the patient is discharged, and ensures that the patient's safety is your top priority.

Option D: This is not ideal as your registrar was not present to review the case with all the information that was available to the consultant during his assessment. There is, however, scope for your registrar to assess the patient himself if it is warranted.

Option H: The physiotherapists are readily available on the ward and are able to make an assessment of the patient's mobility and risk of further falls. Following their assessment, they may advise on additional services that may be required. It is only after an assessment that social services can be involved to arrange packages of care.

Option A: This is not an appropriate course of action. You have justifiable concerns for the patient's welfare and discharge may lead to harm to the patient by omission.

Option C: This is a partially correct answer. While it may be appropriate to involve occupational therapists, you should not directly contact social services before an assessment of the patient's mobility and risk of falls has been completed.

Option E: It may be appropriate to consult the nurses who cater for the daily needs of the patient. However, it would be inappropriate to enact their advice without considering the entire clinical picture or the opinion of the consultant who is ultimately responsible for the patient's care.

Option F: This is not among the best options available. Although you are ensuring that the patient will get assessed for additional support, you are knowingly exposing the patient to potential harm in the interim period between discharge and the assessment.

Option G: This is not an appropriate option. As you are aware that the patient is at risk, you must act promptly. Asking the GP to review will delay an assessment further as he in turn must contact a social worker, which you yourself can instigate prior to discharge. There remains the potential for harm to the patient in the interim period.

Question 13

A, C, B, E, D

When treating a patient, you will commonly find it necessary to maintain a good relationship with their relatives. This can become increasingly difficult when families disagree with both patients and medical teams as to the best course of action. It is important to always act in the patient's best interest and safeguard their autonomy. In this case, it would be advisable to ascertain the patient's capacity to refuse treatment. This option is not available, however. In such circumstances, capacity must be assumed unless demonstrated otherwise. This question does not give cause for concern regarding the patient's capacity.

Option A: This is the most appropriate response, as capacity must be assumed. The patient has the right to refuse treatment and this must be respected. A patient making an inadvisable choice regarding treatment does not constitute a lack of capacity.

Option C: This may be appropriate given the other options available. Senior colleagues may provide insight and support when dealing with requests from the patient's family. They may be in a position to provide advice on further management or assist in difficult consultations involving the patient or their relatives.

Option B: Performing an MMSE will not change the outcome of this situation. An MMSE cannot replace the need for a capacity assessment where required. This option is, however, more suitable than the following options.

Option E: This is an inappropriate answer. By providing treatment, however minimal, you are going against the patient's wishes.

Option D: This is the least appropriate response since treatment is being initiated purely to satisfy the family. You are therefore not acting in the patient's best interest.

Question 14

E, B, C, A, D

Patients have increasing accessibility to information regarding their care through various modes of social media. This presents an additional challenge to the doctor–patient relationship and reaching mutually acceptable management plans. When dealing with an informed patient demanding a drug or investigation, you must attempt to elicit the patient's ideas, concerns and expectations of that particular intervention. Communicating effectively will enable you to understand the reasons for the patient's demands and in turn successfully explain why such a demand is not advisable. When met with such challenges, it is important not to neglect the safeguarding of a patient's welfare and to ensure that you always act in their best interests. These elements should not be sacrificed to appease a patient.

Option E: This is the most appropriate response. By exploring the patient's understanding, using good communication skills, you may be able to deconstruct the misconceptions that are driving the patient to ask for the drug.

Option B: This response is in agreement with GMC guidance on this issue, which states that, should the views of a clinician not agree with those of the patient, a second opinion may be sought. However, this response is not as ideal as the option above, but maintains your integrity as a professional.

Option C: This option is acceptable given that you are preventing unnecessary harm to the patient by prescribing an inappropriate drug that he does not require. By simply refusing, you are not dealing with the underlying reasons for the patient's request and this may have a detrimental effect upon the relationship formed with the patient.

Option A: This is an inappropriate response, as you are unnecessarily prescribing a drug that is not indicated. There is no overall benefit to the patient and it may expose him to the potential adverse effects of the medication.

Option D: This is the least appropriate option, as not only has the drug been prescribed, but there are no plans to review your decision at a later date.

Question 15

B, D, E, A, C

When answering this question, you must first consider whether or not a patient's welfare is put at risk by the registrar's decisions. Making incorrect management plans is of serious concern and could have potentially fatal consequences. Thus in this scenario, you must act quickly to prevent any harm from occurring. Additionally, as with complaints, you must attempt to rectify the problem at a local level, before proceeding to escalate the matter further.

Option B: This is the most appropriate response. By taking the registrar aside, you are dealing with the issue directly and promptly. In a direct conversation, the registrar may justify his actions to you and explain why his plans may be correct. It is also an opportunity for you to flag up your concerns to him, and may avoid the need for further escalation.

Option D: Reporting your concerns to the consultant also deals with the matter directly. If your consultant shares your concerns, he will be able to take action himself to rectify the situation. This is not as ideal as the option above, given that you have escalated your concerns, bypassing the registrar, potentially affecting your relationship with him.

Option E: Contacting a confidential helpline may provide useful advice that is both ethically and legally sound for dealing with this scenario. However, this action does not deal with the situation directly and, in the meantime, the problem remains unresolved with patient safety at risk.

Option A: This response may validate your concerns. It does not, however, attempt to resolve the issue at hand and will not provide any advice on how to progress further. Thus, this option is less suitable than Option E above.

Option C: This response is inappropriate. Patient safety must remain your top priority and your inaction, given your concerns, will potentially place patients at risk.

Question 16

B, D, G

Working in a team involves not only combining individual skills, but also helping other members of that team where possible. In this scenario, the registrar is preparing for an exam and is keen to find time in which she can revise. This is a stressful position to be in and thus you need to demonstrate sympathy to protect your professional relationship. Despite this, patient safety remains paramount, and you need to be aware of your own limitations as well as the competencies of others.

Option B: Refusing the bleep would be an appropriate response. Despite not offering a solution or additional help, it is a suitable answer given the other options available. Accepting the bleep potentially exposes you to dangerous situations, such as an emergency that you are not qualified to deal with. While the registrar will remain on-site, there would be no guarantee that you will be able to contact her at a time of need.

Option D: This is an appropriate response. Suggesting that the bleep is handed over to another registrar would mean suitable equivalent cover for the patients under her care. Your registrar is better placed to make such a request than you are. The registrar in receipt of the bleep can assess whether he or she is able to accept the bleep and provide adequate cover in light of their current clinical workload.

Option G: This is a suitable compromise. You are not accepting the registrar's bleep with its responsibilities, rather you are removing from the registrar some of the responsibilities that you are qualified to handle. Although not a long-term solution, it should provide the registrar with a quiet period in which to revise, while ensuring adequate cover for her patients.

Option A: This is not a suitable option, as you are accepting both the bleep and the responsibilities that it represents. You are neither qualified nor competent to deal with events which require senior attendance.

Furthermore, you may not be able to contact your registrar in the event of an emergency.

Option C: This answer is partially acceptable. Calling the consultant to inform him of the potential for compromised patient care may be necessary. However, making a complaint about your registrar is inappropriate without raising the issue with her first and will adversely affect your professional relationship.

Option E: This is not appropriate, as the librarian is not medically trained and is less suited to judge the importance of the calls received. It is not reasonable to burden the librarian with additional work and place patients at risk of harm.

Option F: This is both inappropriate and unprofessional. Deactivating a bleep prevents important calls from receiving attention, compromising cover and care for patients.

Option H: This response is marginally worse than Option A, given that there is no agreement to contact the registrar if her services are required. The problems of both a lack of suitable cover and working beyond your competencies remain with this answer.

Question 17

D, F, G

This is a very challenging scenario to be faced with, mired in both legal and ethical dilemmas. There are multiple appropriate answers, with some only marginally better than others. The patient's age is key to eliminating some of the inappropriate answers. Given that she is older than 16, capacity to consent to treatment must be assumed, unless a reason to suggest otherwise is given. As with all cases involving minors, there should be a low threshold for involving senior support.

Option D: This is an appropriate response. Exploring the reasons for the request may uncover underlying issues which need addressing before proceeding. Detailing the other options available is necessary to ensure that the patient is making a fully informed decision.

Option F: Asking for senior support is appropriate, given the difficult nature of the case. Experience from a senior member of the team may be required, given the complexity of the patient's decision not to include her parents and the potential legal issues.

Option G: Encouraging the patient to inform her parents is important, despite not having the recourse to tell them yourself. Parental involvement is recommended under GMC guidance. However, if a young adult continues to refuse to involve their parents, you must respect their decision.

Option A: This is inappropriate as it undermines both the relationship with the patient and confidentiality. The patient is assumed to have capacity and this must be respected.

Option B: As an FY1, who is not competent in the procedure or fully registered, you are not able to consent or carry out an abortion. However, given that the patient has capacity, she is able to consent to the treatment without parental knowledge or consent. Before proceeding with an abortion, it would be responsible to explore the patient's situation and inform her of other available options. It would be imperative to involve more senior members of the team who are able to conduct the procedure, and to encourage her to tell her parents.

Option C: Given the patient's age, capacity should be assumed unless there is evidence to suggest otherwise. Only then would a capacity assessment be necessary.

Option E: There are no grounds given in this scenario to refuse the patient's request without further history or investigation.

Option H: Educating the patient about contraception is a preventative measure suited to longer-term management. It does not have an immediate role in this context.

Question 18

C, E, D, A, B

There is continual pressure upon doctors to discharge patients. There is also pressure upon juniors to follow the management decisions of more senior colleagues. It is, however, imperative to ensure that patients are safe and well enough to be discharged. You must stand ready to challenge a decision in the interests of the patient for whom you provide care. In this scenario, both you and a nurse feel that the patient is not suitable for discharge, and as such, you must appropriately escalate your concerns.

Option C: Requesting your registrar to reassess the patient is the most sensible course of action. Given the change in your opinion of the discharge status of the patient, it is not unreasonable to request a repeat review. Your registrar is most apprised of the patient's clinical condition and is most suited to re-evaluate this decision.

Option E: Calling the consultant is the next level of escalation. Bypassing the registrar is not appropriate, but this is a more suitable option than those below.

Option D: Asking another registrar to review the patient may have many implications. It may sour the relationship between yourself and your registrar. Furthermore, you are involving another colleague who is less familiar with the case when there are others who are better placed to review it. This is neither in the patient's interests, nor in keeping with guidance on escalation.

Option A: This response goes against the decision made by a senior doctor. Your registrar's experience may have allowed a more complete assessment of the patient, considering factors that you may have overlooked. In addition, making management decisions that go against the wishes of your senior colleague without consultation is unprofessional. This option is less acceptable than a reassessment of the patient, as a further review may pick up a condition which warrants further treatment, as well as reconfirming a decision to discharge.

Option B: This is an inappropriate response as it potentially puts the patient's safety at risk, particularly given your concerns.

Question 19

E, B, D, A, C

Patients are in a vulnerable position when in hospital and place a measure of trust in their carers. It is important to maintain professionalism when interacting with patients. While rapport is important you must ensure that it is not misinterpreted. However, should a misunderstanding occur, you must endeavour to correct this in a sensitive and reasonable manner. The combination of gratitude and vulnerability on the part of the patient leaves them exposed to potential exploitation. Doctors must ensure that they do not abuse their position of trust to take advantage of others.

Option E: Explaining to the patient the reason why you are unable to maintain a friendship with her is the most appropriate response. The negative response may affect the future doctor–patient relationship; however, the effect is softened by the use of a valid reason. This is the most sensitive approach of the options available.

Option B: Asking for advice from a senior may help to resolve the situation. While their experience will prove helpful, asking them to directly intervene on your behalf is an unnecessary escalation which may prove detrimental. Offloading such a responsibility is not ideal and may further strain the current and future professional relationship you have formed with the patient.

Option D: This is not an ideal response. Maintaining a personal relationship may be perceived as an abuse of your position. Ensuring that she will not be your patient in future is a safeguard against compromising future clinical judgement, but this option still threatens to bring the profession into disrepute as you are taking advantage of the patient's vulnerability.

Option A: Not only are you maintaining a potentially damaging friendship in this option, but you are also failing to ensure the patient's care in future. By allowing this patient to be under your care in the future, you are risking her further care as well as your own clinical judgement by potentially treating a friend.

Option C: This is the least appropriate response. While the above two options compromise professional values and judgement, this response involves lying to the patient, which also compromises your probity.

A, B, E

This scenario involves balancing the patient's confidentiality against acting in her best interests, aiming to reduce the harm to which she is exposed. The situation is a precarious one in which inappropriate actions may further disrupt the relationship and foster further violence on the part of the husband. In keeping with GMC guidance, the 'Good Medical Practice' publication states that 'you must not express to your patients your personal beliefs, including political, religious, or moral beliefs …'. Thus it would not be pertinent to influence the patient in her decision on how to proceed. Giving impartial objective advice is appropriate, allowing the patient to make an informed decision on her course of action.

Central to this question is also the need to protect the patient's confidentiality. She has not given you any grounds to break confidentiality without her consent. This allows you to immediately eliminate a selection of the answers. Breaking confidentiality in this instance could place the patient at risk of further harm.

Option A: Giving the patient information about further action or resources is preferred. You are neither colouring her actions with your opinion, nor are you breaking confidentiality. This option provides her with support and will allow her to obtain expert advice on the matter.

Option B: Asking the advice of a senior colleague would be wise. Given the sensitivity of the situation, the experience of a senior may help you to approach the subject with tact and will validate the advice you eventually offer. Their involvement will help manage and avoid medico-legal issues in this area.

Option E: It is the patient's right to decide whether or not to call the police. You cannot do so on her behalf given that others are not at risk and the patient has not consented to you breaking confidentiality. Offering this advice is correct as the police are trained to deal with domestic abuse cases and may be able to offer further advice and support.

Option C: Arranging to see the husband will inappropriately compromise the patient's confidentiality. Involving the husband may be detrimental to the patient and exacerbate the situation, potentially risking the patient's safety.

Option D: You have no grounds to inform the police given that there is no immediate risk to the patient or other members of the public. In order to make such a disclosure, you would have to obtain the patient's permission.

Option F: Doing nothing is better than breaking confidentiality but is clearly not the best course of action. While your choices are limited, you must attempt to help the patient, even if only by presenting the available options to her.

Option G: This is an inappropriate response. You should not be divulging your subjective personal views to the patient. This option goes against GMC guidance.

Option H: While obtaining a collateral history would be wise given the alcohol history of the patient, it would be best done following consultation with a senior. There may not be a strong suggestion of impaired mental status in the patient and thus approaching a relative would be improper. Furthermore, approaching a relative in cases of impaired mental status would still require you to inform the patient that you intend to break confidentiality.

Question 21

A, B, E

The family in this scenario would clearly like to demonstrate their gratitude with a gift of chocolates. You should approach this question with an initial assessment of the appropriateness of the gift in relation to the level of care you have provided. A box of chocolates is fairly innocuous and is an appropriate gift. There is no suggestion that such a gift may arouse suspicion or be seen to affect the quality of care provided. Declining gifts may potentially be detrimental to the relationship between you and patients or their families. As such, a gift should be declined only if it is out of proportion to the service rendered and this should be done sensitively.

Option A: This is an appropriate response. There is no need to decline such a gift, and you must demonstrate courtesy when accepting it.

Option B: Accepting the chocolates on behalf of the team will help cement the relationship you have with your colleagues, who may have contributed more to the care of the patient than you. Rather than accepting the chocolates on your behalf alone, this will indicate to the family that the gift, or lack of a gift, will not affect your contribution to future care. This will ensure that the gift is less likely to be perceived as a payment for your service.

Option E: Explaining that the gift is not required is a good response. The family will be reassured that they are not under any obligation to impart a gift, in keeping with advice outlined in the GMC publication 'Good Medical Practice' stating that 'you must not encourage patients to give, lend or bequeath money or gifts ...'.

Option C: This option is likely to adversely affect your relationship with the patient's family. Most local procedures do not have blanket policies of refusing gifts. While the guidance is not exhaustive, you must use initiative, and in this circumstance accepting the gift is acceptable.

Option D: While this answer may appear akin to accepting the gift on behalf of the healthcare team, there is a fundamental difference in that asking the nursing staff to intervene is an inappropriate delegation of a task. Since you are aware that the family wish to speak to you, you should endeavour to try to talk to them yourself. Unnecessarily delegating this task may appear rude or discourteous to the family and may affect future relations.

Option F: This answer is a misperception. The gift is appropriate relative to the care provided. Declining the gift on these grounds would be incorrect. Furthermore, this action may adversely affect your relationship with the patient or her family.

Option G: Exploring the reasons may be appropriate if gifts are either recurrent or excessive in nature. Given that this is not the case, it is not necessary to have this conversation with the family.

Option H: There is a key difference between this answer and Option E, whereby the latter was passive in merely informing the family that there is no requirement for a gift, however, this answer is actively discouraging further gifts. Not only is this more likely to cause offence and affect your relationship with the family, but it cannot be supported by the available literature which simply advises against encouraging gifts, but does not endorse discouraging them.

Question 22

E, B, D, A, C

This question combines different aspects of the foundation trainee specification. It is subtly testing your assessment of the situation as well as your understanding of patient safety and maintaining confidentiality. The salient points contained within the question are that it would be very unsafe to send the patient home on oxygen if he is smoking as this is potentially life threatening. However, you must establish the facts before making accusations and acting on your suspicions.

Option E: By talking to the patient in a sensitive manner, you will be able to ascertain whether or not he is truly smoking. The cigarettes in his jacket are merely circumstantial and do not prove anything. By asking the patient out of concern for his safety, it is unlikely that you will threaten the doctor–patient relationship, although maintaining the professional relationship remains secondary to his safety. If the patient denies smoking, this will be an opportunity to counsel him as to the risks of smoking while on home oxygen.

Option B: Escalating the matter to your consultant may offer additional experience and advice in dealing with this further. It is very likely that your consultant will attempt to ascertain the facts by interviewing the patient about your findings. This is, however, an inappropriate escalation given that your personal intervention, as in Option E, is healthier to the doctor–patient relationship and may achieve the same outcome.

Option D: Withdrawing the patient's oxygen may be detrimental to his health and would be an inappropriate response before elucidating the facts as offered in the options above.

Option A: Calling the patient's wife may constitute a breach of confidentiality, particularly if she is unaware that the patient continues to smoke, however, this is an act which is guided by your concerns for the patient's welfare.

Option C: This is the least appropriate response given that you must not cause harm by either act or omission. In this scenario, doing nothing may potentially put the patient's life at serious risk and this is worse than breaking confidentiality.

Question 23

C, B, A, E, D

Patients may refuse to be assessed by particular doctors of the opposite gender on religious or personal grounds. Normal procedure would dictate that you attempt to facilitate the request for a different doctor, however, at times this may not be entirely appropriate or feasible. These testing situations will challenge your general communication and negotiation skills, which you must utilise to attempt to persuade the patient, as well as your improvisation skills to develop a compromise which keeps the patient satisfied.

In a routine situation, there may an opportunity to wait for another doctor of the opposite sex to become available. In this scenario, however, it is clear that time is of the essence, and that the patient's life is at risk. In such situations, the first response would be to safeguard the patient's life by any means possible, but here you are limited by a patient's clear instruction with capacity, that you specifically are not to treat. With this request in mind, the patient has removed the prior justification of implied consent for the action of the intimate exam, in order to save their life. The only time that this request may be disregarded is if the patient has been deemed not to possess the capacity to make this decision, or has demonstrated a reason to suggest as much.

In summary, while the patient should remain your primary concern, the instinct to treat the patient is overruled by the withdrawal of consent, with capacity. In some cases, the patient may refuse to consent to a particular procedure in order to save their life and, as such, you must respect this, but remain aware that you are able to act using other avenues for which the patient has not withdrawn consent. In this complex and challenging scenario, although it is not referenced as an option, you must never neglect input from senior doctors who will better appreciate the case and will be able to provide advice from both a medical and legal viewpoint.

Option C: Looking for a compromise is the best solution to providing the patient with treatment. The compromise could potentially persuade the patient to allow you to proceed, thereby enabling action to save the patient's life with minimal delay. Not only are you prioritising the patient, but you are trying to respect their autonomy.

Option B: Explaining the urgency of the situation and requesting to examine is a good response. It demonstrates that you are keen to prioritise the patient. However, it is subordinate to the option above given that nothing has changed in the situation described in the introduction to the question, and this response lacks any active steps to persuade the patient to reconsider their decision.

Option A: This is an acceptable response which respects the patient's autonomy. However, by waiting for another doctor, you are still neglecting the urgency of the situation and are not being proactive to look for a solution or to attempt to change the patient's mind as in the options above.

Option E: While this response appears attractive at first glance, it involves performing an examination on a patient against their will. They have clearly stated that they do not want you to perform it, and appreciate the gravity of the situation. Even if the patient deteriorates further, the advance decision, with sound mind, means that you cannot perform this examination even if it is in the interests of saving a life.

Option D: This response is inappropriate given that you intend to perform the examination against the patient's will. It is marginally worse than Option E because you are performing the examination more readily, without even giving an opportunity for another doctor to attend before the patient deteriorates.

Question 24

A, B, E

This is a challenging question in which it is important to recognise that, although you are under pressure due to being on-call, you must safeguard the patient's rights. The relative poses a threat to the patient's confidentiality. Not knowing the patient or their preferences means that it would be unwise to divulge any information, without first asking the patient's consent. In addition, there is a limit to the accuracy or amount of information that you can provide, given that this patient is not normally under your care.

Option A: Asking the patient's consent is important before disclosing any information about their care. The patient may not be aware of their relative's request and may not wish to share any sensitive information with her, therefore it would be improper not to establish the patient's wishes first.

Option B: As an FY1 on-call during the weekend, you are responsible for all the patients for whom you provide care. You should thus attempt to answer the questions after gathering information and speaking to the patient to ensure that you have their consent. For more detailed information, the option would remain to inform the relative to speak to the regular medical team. This response will go some way to quell the angry relative and will help to improve the relative's relationship with the patient's regular team.

Option E: The nurses who look after the daily needs of the patient will be well informed of the patient's medical and social progress. They may also be aware of whether the patient has consented to the sharing of information and with whom. Asking the nurses for information does not constitute delegation of responsibility, rather it is an exercise to better prepare you for speaking to the relative yourself.

Option C: This response involves deferring the relative's request to the weekday team. Although the regular team will be better apprised of the situation and be able to offer more accurate and up-to-date information, you have not taken steps to deal directly with the issue at hand. Being on-call for the weekend means that you have a duty of care to the patient, and assume the other responsibilities surrounding that care, including speaking to relatives. Avoiding the conversation is likely to further inflame the situation and make the episode more difficult for the regular team to deal with.

Option D: Your SHO is likely to be busy, and will know no more than you about the circumstances surrounding the patient. This is not a situation that requires senior experience or input and would be an inappropriate escalation.

Option F: This answer is similar to Option C, given that you are not disclosing any information to the relative, however, it is subordinate as you do not offer any alternative or compromise.

Option G: This is an inappropriate response as you have not obtained the patient's permission to disclose any information about them, including that which is written in the handover sheet.

Option H: Calling a colleague outside of their working hours is not advised and should be reserved for urgent matters. This is not a pressing situation which must be dealt with immediately. In addition, your colleague will not have the patient's notes to hand and may be unable to discuss confidential matters due to their location. It should be noted that consultants may commonly call one another on weekends, but each call is made with an appropriate judgement on merit that external input is required. In this case, the matter can easily be deferred to the next working day with little significant consequence and thus does not warrant a call to an off-duty colleague.

Question 25

B, D, G

This scenario is both an ethical and legal predicament to navigate. The question makes clear that the patient's father is a staunch Jehovah's Witness who does not believe in blood transfusion. However, it deliberately evades shedding light on the daughter's beliefs. It is important to remember that she is your patient and you must act in her interests only. In doing this, it would be beneficial to maintain a good relationship with her father, who is the only one available to provide information on her views.

As to the question of where her best interests lie, it is necessary to find out whether she has an advance directive, or whether she is herself a Jehovah's Witness and, if so, whether she has expressed her views on blood transfusions. If such information is impossible to acquire, then her best interests would involve a transfusion to preserve her life before acting to discover this information.

Option B: Questioning the father is the best way to discover whether or not the patient has an advance directive. If so, this would influence further management. It would also facilitate obtaining information on her current beliefs and whether or not they are in conflict with her father's. This is a difficult conversation which must be handled sensitively to obtain the patient's actual views as opposed to projections of what her father believes. Relatives have no legal right to refuse treatment on a patient's behalf in the absence of a signed advance directive.

Option D: Calling a senior colleague is well advised given the potential legal ramifications of this scenario. Senior experience would also prove invaluable in the conversation outlined above. In complex scenarios such as this, you must not neglect senior sanction before acting.

Option G: While this is not the most ideal response, given the paucity of more suitable alternatives, you must act to save the patient's life. Since the patient's religious beliefs and the availability of an advance directive are unclear, it may be necessary to provide a transfusion given the critical status of the patient. Treatment should not progress further than that which is required to sustain her life. At the nearest convenient moment, you would need to take action to obtain consent or confirm the patient's views.

Option A: Giving blood regardless of the patient's views is inappropriate. If the views of the patient are known to any of the healthcare team, they must be honoured. Furthermore, if the patient has expressed her views rejecting a blood transfusion using an advance directive, this is legally binding and must be followed.

Option C: Withholding treatment is inappropriate. Given the seriousness of the patient's condition, and the lack of information, you must act without delay.

Option E: Calling the chaplain may help by providing you with further information regarding how to proceed. This option, however, will further delay lifesaving treatment and is redundant given that the father's consent is not required. As stated above, relatives have no legal right to decline treatment on a patient's behalf.

Option F: This may be an appropriate response if the views of the patient are known in advance. Alternatively, if an advance directive is available, this must be followed. In cases of ambiguity, the patient must be treated first.

Option H: Contacting a religious leader may provide the family with support but does not deal with the situation at hand.

Question 26

C, A, B, D, E

When providing reports to third parties on behalf of patients, you must consider and maintain probity while respecting the patient's confidentiality. GMC guidance published in 'Confidentiality' states that you must 'obtain or have seen written consent to the disclosure from the patient or a person properly authorised to act on the patient's behalf'. Additionally, you must 'only disclose factual information that you can substantiate', and 'offer to show your patient, or give them a copy of, any report that you write about them for employment or insurance purposes before it is sent'. In addition, you must comply with guidance set out in 'Good Medical Practice' ensuring that you:

> ... do your best to make sure that any documents you write or sign are not false or misleading. This means that you must take reasonable steps to verify the information in the documents, and that you must not deliberately leave out relevant information.

The above guidance is particularly concerned with probity and integrity, however, you must ensure that you do not neglect the patient's other rights, including confidentiality. As such, regardless of the content of the report and the initial request to produce it, if the patient demands that the data is not sent, it is your duty to respect this.

Option C: Offering the patient a copy of the report to approve is the action suggested by GMC guidance. Should the patient request that the report is withheld altogether, you would be required to protect his confidentiality.

Option A: When in disagreement with a patient regarding a decision, it is the patient's right to obtain a second opinion. A second opinion is likely to concur with your own and would go some way to reassure your patient that you are acting in the manner expected of a doctor. This option is less likely to affect the professional relationship that you hold with the patient, compared to the option below.

Option B: You are working within the GMC guidance by refusing to send a report which contains falsehoods by omission. However, this response is subordinate to those above, given that a blank refusal without a sensitive approach may sour the relationship that you have with the patient.

Option D: While the patient is acting inappropriately by threatening you with a complaint in order to coerce you into providing a false report, it would be irresponsible to deny further care to the patient on these grounds. GMC guidance states that you must not allow your personal views to affect the treatment of a patient.

Option E: Sending a report containing confidential information against the patient's wishes constitutes a breach of confidentiality. As such, this is the least appropriate response. While Option D is also an inappropriate response, it can be reversed and the implications of denying assistance in this situation are not directly harming the patient. Conversely, submitting the information may adversely affect the patient immediately and harm future prospects of health insurance, even if his blood pressure is brought under control.

Question 27

A, B, E, C, D

There are times when you will find that you elicit information that has eluded other healthcare professionals, including GPs who may not have had the opportunity to obtain such details in time-pressured consultations. When uncovering this information, you must act to remedy the situation. Informing the GP is also important and part of handing over care, but it is necessary to act in the interests of patient care first.

The patient in the scenario has neglected to take his medication because he is forgetful. This may also be because the patient is on a number of different medications, some of which may be unnecessary. Exploring and addressing the reasons why he is not taking his medication may help to remedy the situation. Failing this, informing the GP will allow such issues to be highlighted and followed up in the community. The GP will know the patient better, and may offer an appropriate solution, such as the use of dosette boxes.

Option A: Obtaining an up-to-date list of medication will help you to review the patient's medication more comprehensively. Given the patient's forgetfulness, it is possible that he may be taking medication that has since been stopped, or omitting medication that has recently been started. In the interests of preventing harm from unnecessary medication, it is pertinent to ensure that the patient is taking the correct medication before convincing him to take it regularly.

Option B: Reviewing the medication with the patient addresses one of the reasons why he is not compliant. This will educate the patient on the reasons why he has been prescribed particular drugs, and could convince him to take his medication more regularly. Acting directly in this way will ensure best medical care. While this response does not address the matter of his forgetfulness, it is superior to the other options below.

Option E: Writing a letter to the GP will ensure that the GP is fully informed, and allows for a smooth transition of care back into the community. This will provide the GP with the information that is needed to intervene as necessary and check on the patient to examine whether or not he has begun to take his medication.

Option C: Asking the patient to see his GP is not ideal. You have not taken measures to resolve the situation and are relying on the patient to inform his GP that he is not taking his medication, something he has previously neglected to do. The patient may therefore be lost to follow-up and continue to be poorly compliant, with the resultant adverse effects that this may bring. For this reason, this response is subordinate to Option E. This option also results in you passing on responsibility to other colleagues, when it could more effectively be dealt with by you.

Option D: Giving blank advice to the patient is unlikely to help with the situation. It is likely that the patient knows that he is supposed to take his medication, but is unable to negotiate the obstacles to doing so. This option is less appropriate than Option C, given that the patient's GP is more likely to take positive action.

Question 28

C, D, H

Speaking to bereaved family members is challenging and must be dealt with sensitively. In this scenario, this is exacerbated by the need to convey further bad news at a time of great distress. Such situations present many obstacles and it is important to achieve your objective with minimal collateral damage. You should endeavour to maintain a good relationship with family members, while following whatever protocols are in place.

Team-based care does not end when a patient has died, and continues past death. Thus, you should not hesitate in asking for assistance from both seniors and others who are more experienced in dealing with these matters.

Option C: The patient's father has expressed that his main concern is that his daughter must be buried within 24 hours. Given that a post-mortem must be performed, it is reasonable to explain to him that you will try to arrange it as soon as possible, to allow observance of their religious views. It is important to stress that this cannot be guaranteed; hospital policy on this issue often varies and so this request may not be possible, and the news that it may still be longer than 24 hours should be sensitively broken to the father. This is among the best answers as it directly deals with the father's main concern.

Option D: Interviewing the patient's father may shed light on the reasons for prompt burial or other issues that are central to his disapproval of a post-mortem. This information may prove useful in appeasing the father, and maintaining a good professional relationship with him.

Option H: Bereavement officers are specifically trained in dealing with these types of scenarios and have a wealth of experience, which may include other cases similar to this. They will be fully apprised of hospital policy and protocols which may facilitate the release of the patient's body within 24 hours, should the post-mortem truly be required. While it would be appropriate to approach a senior member of your team regarding complex issues surrounding patients under your care, the bereavement office have the experience to deal with the logistics of such requests. Senior members of your team may be more accustomed to dealing with the medical aspects.

Option A: While this is a good response, it is not among the best answers. Contacting the father's religious leader may clarify the finer points on the acceptability of a post-mortem, and may even offer further guidance on how to make the examination more acceptable. However, contacting a religious leader outside the hospital will infringe upon this imposed

24-hour limit, and will use time that is better spent on first contacting the relevant people within the hospital in order to get the process in motion.

Option B: While the father needs to know that he does not have a choice in this matter, he should be told sensitively and at the appropriate time. Mishandling this piece of information will negatively affect your relationship with the patient's father and potentially his cooperation.

Option E: Other family members may provide support for the patient's father and offer further insight into the situation. While involving other relatives with the father's permission is advised, it is not among the more immediate actions and may serve as a further delay to releasing the patient's body to her family.

Option F: Asking your registrar for advice is a good course of action. It is, however, superseded by the option to approach the bereavement officers, who are better placed to guide you.

Option G: Circumventing the post-mortem by any means would be both unprofessional and a stain upon your probity. While it may be in the interests of the family, it may not be in the interests of the patient, who is your primary concern.

Question 29

E, B, C, A, D

It is important to balance the many issues that are involved in this question. First and foremost, you must identify that there is potential for harm to patients given that the nurse has sustained a needle-stick injury. Concurrently, this must be weighed against the nurse's own welfare and right to confidentiality. Acting inappropriately may impact on your relationship with the nurse in question.

While needle-stick injuries have the potential to transfer a variety of pathogens, the most concerning would be the transmission of hepatitis B virus, hepatitis C virus and Human Immunodeficiency Virus (HIV). Guidance published in 'HIV Infected Health Care Workers: Guidance on Management and Patient Notification' by the Department of Health states:

> A healthcare worker who has any reason to believe they may have been exposed to infection with HIV, in whatever circumstances, must promptly seek and follow confidential professional advice on whether they should be tested for HIV. Failure to do so may breach the duty of care to patients.

Further guidance suggests that those who suspect that they may have been exposed to HIV should ensure that 'procedures which are thought to be exposure prone must not be performed whilst expert advice is sought'. The document also reminds all healthcare workers that where you are aware of the health status of another member of staff, that 'there is a duty to keep such information confidential'.

Option E: This is the most appropriate response. Patient safety is the primary concern and must be safeguarded. This option is preferred to Option B, for this purpose alone. Although the nurse may have been exposed to a communicable disease, this does not limit them from working with patients, with the exception that they must not perform risky procedures during the time when such a disease is suspected.

Option B: Guidance from the Department of Health requires that the nurse must immediately seek professional advice with regards to this exposure. As such, this is a high-priority response that is superseded only by GMC guidance that safeguarding patients should remain the first priority.

Option C: Calling the patient to obtain a sample of their blood may prove to be of some benefit. However, this is better left for occupational health to do, given that they are better trained in these matters and may be able to safeguard the nurse's identity.

Option A: This is an immediate action which should have been undertaken at the time of the injury. It is now of little benefit, and does not rank highly given the time that has passed since the event.

Option D: This is the least appropriate response. The events which have transpired do not require the submission of an incident form given that a patient did not suffer and was not at risk of harm. Completing an incident form needlessly risks revealing the nurse's identity and will damage your working relationship with the nurse. This is less appropriate than Option A given the additional potential to exacerbate the situation.

Question 30

E, A, B, D, C

Most smokers do attempt to give up smoking with limited success. Not all of them present to a doctor with such a complaint, but occasional screening with a simple question of whether they would like assistance to quit can be quite revealing. Although this question pertains specifically to smoking, the principles that it tests relate more to assessing a situation, weighing up the evidence and not being prejudiced towards a patient due to their actions or beliefs.

Abandoning smoking is in the patient's best interests, and will promote better health. Acting in the patient's interests means that you should provide her with the necessary help to quit. This is part of placing your patient as your first priority. Thus, it is clear that you should provide an intervention. The information you have been given can partially guide you towards a course of action, and tells you that certain interventions have not previously worked. It is therefore evident that you must consider alternatives.

Option E: Discussing the patient's previous attempts and problems would be very useful. Smoking is a lifestyle choice as opposed to a disease, and is thus facilitated by other factors such as stress. Furthermore, identifying problems with previous attempts and interventions will help to select a more suitable intervention than blindly selecting an alternative to patches. By talking to the patient, you may also be able to further motivate the patient which may prove very effective in getting the patient to quit.

Option A: Considering alternatives to patches is appropriate in this scenario. Patches have not worked in the past and the patient is clearly motivated to quit. They may not have worked because of improper use or because she is not amenable to them. Giving patches where other options are available may be a waste of resources and the patient's time.

Option B: While prescribing patches is an attempt to help the patient give up smoking, it is not a good answer in light of the options above.

Option D: Not providing an intervention, even patches, is insensitive and inappropriate. The patient would benefit from an intervention, and has expressed motivation to quit. Providing an intervention will improve the patient's chances of abstinence.

Option C: Simply insisting that the patient avoids smoking is inappropriate. The aim of intervention is to aid in abstinence. If the patient has failed to stop in the past with patches, the likelihood of abstinence without intervention is very unlikely. This in effect means that you are not helping the patient at all. This response is therefore subordinate to Option D, given that you have imposed a condition upon further treatment and have in fact introduced another obstacle to the patient giving up smoking.

Question 31

A, D, E, B, C

Maintaining relationships with your colleagues is important and useful when arranging exchanges of on-call shifts. In this scenario, you have caught another FY1 conducting a disciplinable offence. While you may feel a moral obligation to flag up your discovery, you must ensure to escalate this sensitively. Approaching this without tact may affect not only your relationship with the FY1, but also the FY1's relationship with other colleagues, as they may resent having to cover someone who has feigned illness.

Option A: Talking to your colleague in the first instance would be wise. You are taking action designed to prevent a recurrence, and have informed your colleague of your intention to escalate if his behaviour continues. This action allows for the FY1 to make amends or explain himself and may be as effective as disciplinary action by a senior without compromising his relationship with you or the other FY1s.

Option D: Discussing this incident with your team will limit the amount of people who are aware of the incident and the prospect of disciplinary action against the FY1 in question, protecting your relationship with him. The experience of your SHO may give valuable guidance on how to proceed and what action to take. It may even help to protect the identity of the FY1 and allude to hypothetical scenarios. The involvement of others in this matter, however, makes this option less preferential to Option A.

Option E: Informing your consultant is a significant step. By informing a person in a position of responsibility, you may ensure that the matter is addressed. However, this is in fact escalating the situation and may negatively affect your relationship with the FY1. The outcome of the escalation in reference to the FY1's conduct is likely to be the same with the addition of repercussions compared to you handling the situation alone or with advice. Thus this option is subordinate to those above.

Option B: Ignoring what you have seen is an inadequate action. You have witnessed a colleague doing something wrong and must address it or at least make them aware that it is inappropriate. Not doing anything while patient care is potentially put at risk is unbecoming of a doctor.

Option C: Asking for a bribe is both unprofessional and unethical. This is the least appropriate answer given that you are undertaking immoral behaviour yourself.

Question 32

C, B, A, D, E

Flagging up issues pertaining to your consultant can be very difficult as this challenges the hierarchical respect that you hold for them. It is made even more so given that your team does not seem to have noticed these issues and are not validating your concerns. Despite the complexity of the situation, you must identify the potential to compromise patient care and take active measures to prevent this.

When approaching this situation, care needs to be taken in order to preserve the working relationship you have with both your consultant and the rest of the team. While whistleblowing is generally looked upon negatively, it must not be neglected when required. Sensitivity, however, is necessary when assessing a situation to gauge whether such rash action is required. This scenario highlights a deterioration in your consultant's appearance which may be a sign of greater neglect. You have a duty towards your consultant to establish the facts and protect patients through appropriate escalation rather than drastic action, which may be out of proportion to the gravity of the situation.

Option C: Approaching your colleagues provides two distinct advantages over the other options. Firstly, it will validate your concerns and confirm whether your observations are in fact noteworthy rather than an over-evaluation of a harmless situation. Secondly, your colleagues may be able to offer advice on how to proceed. Advice from senior colleagues would be preferred in this case as they are privy to the same information as you, and will be able to call upon their greater experience.

Option B: Asking to speak to your consultant is a good response. Although there is a risk of causing offence or harming your professional relationship, these risks must be accepted as patient safety must be safeguarded at all costs. However, by approaching the matter sensitively and respectfully, such outcomes can be avoided. This option directly addresses the subject of patient safety and limits the circle of individuals who are aware of the problem, but should be preceded by Option C to ensure that such action is warranted.

Option A: Asking your peers for advice is not advised. It is unlikely that they will have the experience to deal with such matters and this action may compromise the confidentiality of the situation. It fails to deal with the matter of patient safety, and could adversely affect your relationship with the team.

Option D: This is an unnecessary escalation and is not a suitable course of action. However, this response is preferred to Option E given that notifying the GMC is a measure that is undertaken to limit harm to patients.

Option E: Ignoring your observations may be negligent if you suspect a risk to patients. This answer is the least appropriate.

Question 33

C, D, B, A, E

Events such as that outlined in the question are fortunately rare. However, mistakes still do happen and the consequences can be very severe. Guidance published in 'Good Medical Practice' states:

> If a patient under your care has suffered harm or distress, you must act immediately to put matters right, if that is possible. You should offer an apology and explain fully and promptly to the patient what has happened, and the likely short-term and long-term effects.

In this scenario, you must keenly identify that not only has your patient received expired medication, but that there is the possibility that other patients are at risk of the same experience. Before taking rash action that may cause panic or unduly upset patients, it is reasonable to verify facts. After addressing the immediate aspects of this case, it is then necessary to take measures to prevent incidents from recurring.

Option C: Checking the bag against the drug chart will help to ascertain whether indeed the patient has received the expired saline bag in question. There may exist an innocuous reason for which the expired saline remained near the patient, such as identification by the nurse as unsuitable for use. Before raising the alarm about this incident, it would be wise to verify the facts, given that a false alarm would unnecessarily distress the patient and other patients and may adversely affect the doctor–patient relationship.

Option D: Raising the incident with the ward manager would give them an opportunity to check the other saline bags in stock and ensure that they are not polluted with expired bags. Additionally, the ward manager may action the nurse to check the fluids being received by the other patients to ensure their safety.

Option B: It is important to notify the patient promptly when an error has occurred and to outline to them the risks and potential outcomes that may result from the mistake. This is superseded by Option D, due to the prospect of harm to patients that could be prevented, as opposed to explaining harm that has already occurred.

Option A: Given that this scenario involves direct harm to a patient, you are obligated to complete an incident form, and to inform the patient. The purpose of the incident form is to investigate the cause of the error and to prevent it in future. While important, it is crucial to complete more pressing actions first, such as informing the patient.

Option E: Even though it is correct to document the incident in the notes, concealing the event from the patient is inappropriate and contravenes guidance. For this reason, this is the least appropriate response.

Question 34

B, E, H

Approaching a radiologist for requests can be a daunting task for a newly qualified doctor. Slots for procedures tend to be limited and it is therefore imperative that patients are prepared ahead of their allocated time. With interventional requests an INR <1.3 is ideal, however, some radiologists may accept INRs of up to 1.5 in exceptional cases. This requirement is related to safeguarding patients from the risks of the procedure. Good communication with the radiologists and your team are imperative to ensure that you are clear on the reasons why a procedure is necessary and its importance in influencing the patient's further management.

Radiologists commonly have a reputation for brevity and being meticulous, which comes with the territory of guarding a limited resource against the entire hospital. When precious slots are wasted due to inadequate preparation, it is understandable for a radiologist to be aggrieved and express the magnitude of their annoyance by refusing to perform the procedure at all. This, however, is not a reason to avoid the radiologist, but an opportunity to provide or request solutions in the interest of your patient who must remain your first priority.

Option B: Approaching the radiologist a second time with the patient fully prepared may appease him sufficiently in order to agree to perform the procedure. Expressing the urgency if appropriate may prompt him to schedule the patient as early as possible.

Option E: Explaining that you have tried unsuccessfully to prepare the patient for the procedure may allow you to discuss further options with the radiologist, who may be able to use his experience to suggest alternatives. It may not be in the patient's best interests to have the liver biopsy in light of the raised INR and other measures may require discussion.

Option H: Discussing with your seniors about the importance of the biopsy may govern the next step in the patient's management. If it is indeed urgent, your registrar may offer alternative measures for preparing the patient for the procedure and may opt to speak to the radiologist directly to discuss the patient's case in more detail.

Option A: The radiologist has valid reasons to justify their actions. Excessively escalating the issue to the GMC is therefore not appropriate.

Option C: Interrupting your consultant at a time when he is busy and his advice is not urgently required, given that the patient has missed his slot and other senior team members are available, is not advised. Escalating the situation to your consultant can wait, as no immediate action can be taken. Your registrar is in a suitable position to advise you in the interim.

Option D: Complaining to another colleague about your perceived negative experience is unprofessional and will affect your working relationship, potentially with both radiologists. This is not advised, especially since you will undoubtedly have to continue working closely with them in the future.

Option F: While it may be appropriate to apologise to the radiologist, this response does not directly resolve the problem of having a patient who is not adequately prepared for the procedure. This response is therefore subordinate to Options B and E, where active measures are being undertaken to address the problem. Asking the radiologist to circumvent protocol by performing the procedure is not in the best interests of the patient.

Option G: Undermining the on-call radiologist's authority by attempting to by-pass him is unprofessional. Before approaching another radiologist who is not necessarily on-call, it would be wise to explore the other available options, as stated above. This would, however, be an appropriate response, should the on-call radiologist continue to decline to perform the procedure despite a corrected INR, but it remains superseded by the options above.

Question 35

A, C, G

You must be fully competent in a procedure, before performing it independently. If not, it must be performed under supervision. It is clear from the scenario that you have only watched the procedure once in a controlled environment and you can therefore conclude that you are not competent at performing it on a patient without supervision. Given that the procedure itself is elective and not an emergency, you do not have the justification to attempt it without adequate training.

The challenges posed by the scenario include preserving the doctor–patient partnership as well as safeguarding your own professionalism. The patient will undoubtedly be very dissatisfied with the prospect of waiting for a service that is not going to happen, but this is secondary to compromising her safety by attempting it. Furthermore, you should aim to limit the patient's dissatisfaction through other available means.

Option A: While inserting the device with supervision would be ideal, this is not an option. If insertion is not possible on a given day, it would be appropriate to provide the patient with another appointment, and to offer interim temporary contraception for protection in the meantime.

Option C: Calling your supervising GP is advisable. They will be able to inform you whether or not they are likely to come back soon and, if so, whether there is a chance that the procedure will happen or not. Given this information, you will be able to advise and provide options to the patient. If the procedure is possible on the day, this will allow the patient to choose to wait or arrange another appointment.

Option G: Although asking another senior is not the most ideal solution, it allows for the patient to leave with the intrauterine device in place. The option does specify that the other senior is suitable to supervise and willing to do so, thus this option is also feasible.

Option B: This response is inaccurate. Judging yourself to be competent given the description in the question is not correct, and it would therefore be inappropriate to perform the procedure without adequate supervision.

Option D: Keeping the patient waiting in the room is not a good response. There is no guarantee that the GP will return soon, and even if he does, he may not be able to supervise that day. Keeping the patient waiting needlessly before telling her that the procedure will not happen will have a greater negative impact on the doctor–patient relationship.

Option E: Asking the GP to instruct you over the phone will not help to make the procedure safer. Over the phone, the GP will not be able to watch to ensure that you are performing the procedure correctly. Furthermore, should any complications arise, the GP will not be present to identify them or intervene.

Option F: This is a good response but it is subordinate to other available options. In this answer, you have identified that you are not competent or able to conduct the procedure, and are willing to rebook the patient. However, this answer ranks below Option A because there is no offer to provide interim measures, which are important in this scenario.

Option H: Asking the patient whether or not she is willing to wait presents a caveat. Should the patient choose to stay, there is no indication that the GP will arrive at a reasonable hour, and if he does, there is no certainty that he will have the time to supervise you or indeed perform the procedure himself.

Question 36

E, C, B, D, A

This is a commonly tested scenario that is very challenging. There are three elements to be considered here. Firstly, is it appropriate to break confidentiality and, before doing so, have you given the patient enough opportunity to disclose the issue himself? Secondly, is the public interest sufficient to warrant breaking confidentiality? And thirdly, are you escalating the situation correctly and at the appropriate time? Among these considerations, you must also pay attention to the effect that your actions will have on the relationship that you have built with the patient.

The guidance on breaking confidentiality has been reviewed in earlier chapters. In summary, it is important to try and persuade the patient to inform his wife of his own volition. Failing that, if there is a significant risk of public harm, you probably do have grounds to break confidentiality. Before taking such an irreversible step, it is advisable to involve a senior to validate your actions. Finally, before taking such an action, you should inform the patient that you are going to break confidentiality, and to whom. During these types of cases, the importance of proper documentation cannot be over emphasised.

Option E: This is the best option. If you manage to persuade the patient to inform his family himself, you will not have to break confidentiality and will avoid the complications and legal risks associated with it.

Option C: Given the complexity and legal ramifications of alternate options in this scenario, involving seniors early on is recommended. A consultant will draw on their experience and offer good advice in addition to doublechecking your groundwork to ensure that your actions are legally sound.

Option B: Informing the patient that he must tell his wife, or you will do so, gives the patient the opportunity to act. As you are threatening to break confidentiality, it is preferred to involve the consultant as in the option above. Breaking confidentiality is irrevocable and should be done with a consultant's approval wherever possible.

Option D: This is a necessary step before proceeding with actually breaking confidentiality. This response is subordinate to Option B given that this action is implied in Option B which also offers the addition of allowing the patient the opportunity to resolve the situation himself.

Option A: Doing nothing is unacceptable. There is obvious risk to another individual and the public interest weighs very heavily here. Not acting at all would be negligent and wholly inappropriate.

Question 37

B, G, H

The arrival of foreign patients in A&E prompts difficulties in management and follow-up. The publication 'Good Medical Practice' states that, 'in an emergency, wherever it arises, you must offer assistance', with aftercare and ongoing management remaining a grey area which may be subject to local policy. You therefore have a duty to manage the acute problem that the patient presents with, although this does not necessarily extend to longer-term care. Although discriminating against patients would be unethical and potentially illegal, treating a foreign patient fully, as you would a UK national, may land the patient with a large bill that he is unable to afford. The key to this question is identifying that the patient is acutely unwell and requiring urgent medical attention, which must therefore be provided.

Option B: In addition to treating the acute symptoms, telling the patient to return if his symptoms come back is normal safety net advice. This should always be offered to any patient. Should this patient return in an emergency, he would be treated immediately until he is stable.

Option G: The patient has come in with an acute emergency. You must treat him immediately and provide symptomatic relief, though further management is less appropriate in this scenario as the patient will be responsible for the expenses. This response is superior to Option F because no prescription is offered, which is better than discharging the patient with an NHS prescription to which he may not be entitled.

Option H: Asking the registrar for advice is very important. Further action beyond urgent treatment is likely to be subject to local policy, as it may compromise the Trust.

Option A: While you may be correct in refusing to prescribe the inhaler, this option is subordinate to those above, given that it does not acknowledge that the patient requires urgent treatment first.

Option C: This is a good response that must be completed. Once the patient is treated, he will require follow-up, the prerequisite of which is an adequate handover. This answer does not figure in the top three, as it is not as pressing as urgent treatment.

Option D: Refusing treatment is ethically and morally wrong in such circumstances. This is an inappropriate response.

Option E: This answer is inaccurate. The patient does have the right to urgent treatment, given the seriousness of his presenting complaint. In reference to obtaining replacements for his lost inhalers, this is not an emergency and the patient will require a private prescription. However, you are not obligated to provide this.

Option F: Treating the patient for his asthma would be appropriate. Writing the NHS prescription for his inhalers, however, may be against protocol. Thus, in light of a better alternative above, this response is not among the correct answers.

Question 38

D, A, E, B, C

Pain is an incredibly subjective phenomenon. While attempts can be made to measure it, none have really proven to be infallible. Thus, one of the best guides is in fact the patient experiencing the pain and the information that they provide you with.

In this scenario, the question is hinting at the idea that the patient is exhibiting drug-seeking behaviour. It is a very precarious situation in which you must weigh the harm of your potential actions. Put simply, you can either provide or refuse to provide analgesia. Supplying the additional medication may be facilitating an addiction and indirectly causing harm to the patient. There is also the danger of overdosing the patient. On the other hand, refusing the medication may cause the patient pain and be harming the patient through omission. Given that different people experience pain differently, even if your patient appears well, they may in fact be in need of analgesia. Due to the fact that leaving the patient in pain is worse than overtreating pain, it is generally better to provide the smallest amount of analgesia possible in these circumstances, rather than to deny it altogether. With this approach, you are likely to cause the least harm.

Option D: Obtaining a brief history will shed light on the situation. Asking the right questions, you may be able to ascertain whether there are other alternatives to analgesia, whether it can be avoided altogether, or maybe what amount to prescribe. This should be the first thing to do as it will supplement and guide your prescribing.

Option A: Since the patient is complaining of pain, you need to do something about it. Although you may suspect that you are fuelling an addiction, you cannot definitively say the patient is without pain. Although this is less ideal than offering a non-analgesic alternative, it is the only option available that offers positive action against the pain. It would be advisable to prescribe the smallest dose possible. This option is subordinate to Option D, given that Option D is performed with a view to providing treatment.

Option E: Given the difficulty of the situation, it would be reasonable to request help from your SHO. This response ranks third as your SHO will be in the same position as yourself and will need to provide analgesia or a suitable alternative to tide the patient over until morning. Although they have greater experience to draw on when considering management options, they will essentially do what you would do, but may have greater experience to advise you and manage the situation accordingly.

Option B: Recording observations and writing a recommendation is important but does not deal with the patient's pain. It may be a form of legal protection to suggest that you saw the patient to ensure their condition was not life threatening, but the fact remains that the patient is still in pain.

Option C: Denying the patient analgesia without recourse to an alternative is inappropriate. Even though the patient may be abusing medication, your assessment may be incorrect and they may truly be in pain. It is safer to overprescribe a small amount than to deny help to a patient in pain. The patient's regular team can reassess the situation in the morning.

Question 39

A, B, C

This scenario is an emergency in which you need to act quickly to save the patient's life. It is quite clear that you are unaware of how to use the support which is required to prevent the patient from bleeding, and are thus not competent in its application. Doing so without adequate guidance may worsen the patient's clinical condition. Given the nature of the situation and the patient's dependence upon this equipment, it would thus be acceptable to attempt to fit the support with guidance that would normally be deemed to be insufficient.

Option A: You have sufficient training to manage this patient supportively. This will provide a larger window for help to arrive and apply the pelvic support.

Option B: While not ideal, applying the support is paramount to the survival of the patient. Guidance over the phone would not be acceptable in non-urgent scenarios. However, the benefits of this outweigh the potential drawbacks. The consultant is available over the phone and given the urgency of the situation, it will be beneficial to utilise this resource.

Option C: Providing details of this patient to your other seniors will allow them to reassess and reprioritise their commitments. Asking the nurse to relay the information allows you to remain with the patient and continue with life-saving measures.

Option D: This is a good response. Bleeping the ward team could be useful given their experience. Despite this, they may not respond and may be attending to urgent matters or theatres themselves. They are under no obligation to help you given that they are not on-call, but may help out of professional courtesy.

Option E: Informing the senior team members may alert them to the magnitude of the emergency with which you are dealing. However, it is unwise to visit them yourself and leave the patient unattended at such a critical moment. This action is compromising the patient's care.

Option F: Calling the patient's family is an important task that should be completed later when the patient is stable and not in need of immediate management.

Option G: Calling the crash team may be appropriate if the patient is in arrest or peri-arrest. This is not the case and tying up the crash team for this patient may delay their attendance to a more urgent genuine crash call.

Option H: Attempting to fit the support without training or guidance may be detrimental and worsen the patient's condition, particularly if his garments are supporting his pelvis. Applying the support incorrectly may contribute to the patient's deterioration.

Question 40

C, D, B, A, E

Patients refusing procedures to which they have previously consented is a source of frustration for the already stretched junior doctor. Nonetheless, patients retain the right to refuse and their decisions must be appreciated.

Capacity should be assumed in these scenarios, however, there is no harm in confirming that the patient has capacity, and should capacity be present or absent, the result should be documented in the notes. With an elderly lady who has been suffering from iron-deficiency anaemia, there is a good possibility of an active gastrointestinal bleed and the ensuing anaemia is a plausible cause of an acute loss of capacity. One should also not neglect infection in such episodes. This makes a capacity assessment all the more important.

Additionally integrated into this question are considerations concerning confidentiality and best interests. In simple terms, confidentiality should not be broken without permission and at least prior notification. In the case of diminished capacity, it is assumed that the patient would permit the breaking of confidentiality to discuss their best interests with the next of kin, if capacity was intact. Furthermore, best interests do not require discussion until a lack of capacity has been established.

Option C: This is the best response. A quick capacity assessment would be ideal to establish whether the patient is able to make the decision to refuse treatment. Indirectly, you would uncover the patient's insight into the outcome of refusing the treatment. Whatever the outcome of the assessment, the result should be documented in the notes, as it contributes to medico-legal defence in the case of a bad outcome.

Option D: This response would give an idea as to the extent of the patient's insight. It is incorporated in Option C, which constitutes a fuller assessment. Should the patient not have insight, it would be a cue to conduct a formal capacity assessment and to consider acting in the patient's best interests with senior input.

Option B: Respecting the patient's wishes is the default response. In accordance with the law, as reviewed in earlier chapters, you should assume capacity unless there is evidence otherwise. It is better not to perform the procedure, than to coerce the patient into it without proving a lack of capacity and thus acting in the patient's best interests.

Option A: Phoning the patient's family to confirm her best interests would require disproving capacity first, and thus may be an inappropriate action. There is also a risk that you are inappropriately breaking confidentiality by calling the family without consulting the patient. This action is ranked above Option E because it is not as drastic as performing a procedure against a patient's will when you have not proven that patient is unable to decide.

Option E: This option is inappropriate given that you do not have consent for the procedure. Furthermore, capacity must be assumed in this response as there is no definitive evidence or proof that she lacks it.

Question 41

E, D, C, B, A

It is a professional duty to ensure proper handover and to provide adequate cover during and between on-call shifts. After a long and weary on-call with only ten minutes to go, it is very easy to neglect your bleep and hand over these calls to your successor. However, if bleeps arrive before the start of the next shift, even if it is during handover, they are your responsibility to respond to. While this is the official stance, camaraderie between colleagues may mean your successor will offer to respond to the call on your behalf.

Nurses may bleep you with a variety of requests; some may be urgent, bordering upon emergencies, while others may be inappropriate. Regardless of the diversity, it is your job to sort through these calls and attend to them according to priority. As such, it is good practice to respond to your bleeps promptly, if only to assess.

Option E: This is the ideal response. If the call is an emergency, then you must act quickly to ensure patient safety. If, however, the call is routine and can wait, it may be better to ensure a proper handover in which you also hand over the new job for your colleague to complete.

Option D: It is better to blindly deal with a bleep than to hold it off until later given the chance that the call is in fact an emergency. This action is conducive to maintaining patient safety.

Option C: Answering the bleep and deferring it until later is not ideal. Without assessing the request, you have no idea whether or not it is urgent. Should the call be urgent, it would be more important to attend to it than handing over to your colleague.

Option B: Neither Option B nor Option A are appropriate responses, as both involve ignoring the bleep until after handover. The bleep could potentially be an urgent request that requires immediate attention. Option B is, however, preferred, given that your colleague has just begun his shift, while your shift is ending. This is especially so if the request is something that requires a lot of time to deal with, which would impact on your work/life balance. While in most instances it is advisable that you avoid passing responsibility over to a colleague with something that you could deal with, in this instance the possibility that you may stay excessively past your allotted time makes Option B the preferred response.

Option A: This answer is the least appropriate. It is marginally worse than the option above as it impinges on your work/life balance. Assessing the call after handover will mean that you will overstay at the hospital following your shift. Ideally, calls which you cannot attend to on time and which are not urgent should be handed over; the bleep arrived on your shift and thus you have a professional responsibility to answer it, as it is part of the cover that you provide. It is sensible to hand over this request, and make this clear to the nurse that has contacted you.

Question 42

C, E, D, B, A

This scenario broaches the subject of disapproval of the decisions made by seniors. The description highlights that you are uncomfortable with the choices that your consultant is making, particularly as they go against recommended guidelines. With patient safety as your priority, it is appropriate to raise your concerns and take the necessary steps to safeguard them. When challenging a senior, you must do so sensitively, and appreciate that guidelines are suggestions that require interpretation, from which deviation may be required in particular cases.

Option C: Exploring your consultant's decisions may be interpreted as a challenge to his decision. However, if approached in the correct manner, it can serve as a learning point to educate you in the specific management of patients with particular complaints and presentations. Going directly to the consultant will give the most accurate information, without compromising their authority.

Option E: The registrar will also be familiar with the patients and may be aware of the reasons behind the consultant's decisions. This can again be seen as an educational point rather than a challenge to the consultant's authority. This is subordinate to Option C because you are involving another party instead of speaking to the person who is responsible for the decision and can justify it best.

Option D: A literature review may uncover the reasons for the decisions from the latest evidence. However, information from literature is not case specific, and may need further expert interpretation before application to your patients. This response is preferred to the options below as it does not undermine your consultant's authority and compromise your professional relationship with them.

Option B: Speaking to another consultant may validate your concerns. However, escalating the matter ahead of your team is not preferred in light of the other options and may affect your working relationship with your consultant. The other consultant may not be familiar with the patients under your care and so would be unable to provide accurate reasoning for your consultant's decisions.

Option A: Notifying the GMC is an inappropriate escalation given that you have not explored the reasons behind your consultant's decisions or confirmed that patients have been put at risk.

Question 43

E, G, H

Negotiating with patients is made all the more difficult when they present armed with medical knowledge. This scenario is complicated by the fact that your patient is a foreign doctor who is accustomed to a policy that varies from the one employed by your hospital. Furthermore, there is no information on the country in which he developed his pneumonia, which is crucial to deciding upon the appropriate selection of antibiotics. Local policy tends to apply to locally contracted pneumonia and thus the patient may have sufficient grounds for his request. While it is important to follow hospital guidelines, there is room to employ both clinical judgement and initiative. With additional information from the patient, it may be necessary to heed his request and deviate from the guidelines, but you should not hesitate to seek senior approval before doing so.

Option E: Taking a detailed history is paramount to the correct selection of antibiotics. Ascertaining the country and timing of the onset of symptoms will assist in choosing to adhere or deviate from the guidelines and is information that will be requested by your seniors and microbiology colleagues.

Option G: Calling the microbiologist is advisable since they are the experts on infections and antimicrobial selection, and will be acquainted with antibiotic guidelines. When there is a case for deviating from hospital policy, it is prudent to inform them and seek their advice on the most appropriate antibiotics.

Option H: It is common practice to treat infections empirically until the correct antibiotics are identified by sensitivities from culture results. Explaining this to the patient is important and is a compromise to his demands, which may still be met. It is appropriate to treat the patient in keeping with local policy given that you do not currently possess conclusive evidence to justify a different selection.

Option A: Hospital policies tend to be guidelines as opposed to rigid rules which must be followed. An element of initiative should be used when interpreting guidelines. In this scenario, there may be a case for deviating from policy given that the infection may not be local.

Option B: Prescribing antibiotics inappropriately is poor practice that promotes antibiotic resistance. Selection must always be corroborated by clinical evidence which is lacking for the use of both sets of antibiotics.

Option C: Asking senior advice is appropriate but is superseded by the option of involving the microbiologists who are in a better position to advise you on the choice of antibiotics. Your registrar is likely to direct you towards Options G and H, and thus consulting with them is an obsolete response.

Option D: This response is based on an assumption that the pneumonia was acquired from the patient's native country. The question does not provide the evidence to support this and you must therefore treat empirically and await sensitivities.

Option F: This may be an appropriate response, however, deterioration of the patient does not conclusively prove that the antibiotic selection is incorrect. This is superseded by culture results which provide a better quality of evidence to adjust antibiotic therapy.

Question 44

E, A, B, D, C

Competently negotiating with patients and their families is an important communication skill. In an age where a wealth of information is available on the internet, patients are more likely to present armed with knowledge and specific requests. It is part of your vocation to continue to educate the patient and to explain the rationale for requesting or refusing specific investigations.

As a first response, before any affirmative action, it is important to gather as much information from your patient as possible. While doing this, building rapport is essential, and will be useful in the case of refusing a request. Documentation in these circumstances is important, not least given the possibility of a complaint following a perceived unfavourable outcome on behalf of the patient.

Option E: Obtaining a medical history will help you to narrow down the cause of the patient's headaches and to treat them effectively. Using the history to guide you, you can ascertain whether a CT scan is indicated and if it is not, you will be able to justify your decision. This also allows you to then respond with confidence to the mother's concerns and reassure her that a CT scan is not indicated after ruling out red flags from the history you elicited.

Option A: Discussing ideas, concerns and expectations with the mother will help to direct the conversation. Her request for a CT scan is probably borne out of a deep-seated concern for a specific pathology. Eliciting these concerns will allow you to better help her understand that a CT scan is not in the interests of her son. This should be done once a complete history has been elicited.

Option B: While this statement may be true, it is not a sensitive way to break the news to the mother, and gathering further information is preferred before making such statements. Blindly telling the mother that a scan is not ideal does not provide any justification, nor does it address her concerns. Breaking this news to her after all the appropriate information has been gathered, allows you to confidently justify your decision.

Option D: Documentation is very important. This is a legal record of your actions and justifications. Despite its importance, it should be prioritised after interacting with the patient and his family.

Option C: Prescribing analgesia is the last priority in this scenario. The patient is not in pain and does not currently require medication. Your immediate action should be to address the concerns of the patient and his mother, for which she has approached you. This option would have ranked higher as a more appropriate answer if the patient was currently in pain.

Question 45

E, A, B, D, C

When confronted by a clinical situation that challenges your moral or religious views, it is important to be honest about these as they may impact on the care that you provide. The GMC publication 'Good Medical Practice' states that, in instances where patient care may be compromised due to your religious or moral beliefs, '… you must explain this to the patient and tell them they have the right to see another doctor', and '… you must ensure that arrangements are made for another suitably qualified colleague to take over your role'. You should remain non-judgemental in your practice and not discriminate against your patients based on their life choices and beliefs. If this is not practical, a suitably qualified colleague should attend to the patient in your place. Where this is not possible, you should see the patient yourself, following the guidance above.

Option E: Asking the SHO to see the patient allows for an unbiased clinician to review and prescribe analgesia accordingly. While this inconveniences your colleague, this is an appropriate escalation as your position is compromised and your SHO should be your next port of call.

Option A: Requesting that the anaesthetist reviews the patient ensures an objective opinion on the patient. While the anaesthetist is the appropriate expert, this matter is under your remit and as such, the SHO should be called before leaving the chain of escalation.

Option B: If there are no other colleagues who are available to see the patient, you should review the patient yourself. In accordance with guidance, you must inform the patient of your subjectivity and offer the choice of a second opinion in place of your own. This response is less appropriate than those above as it potentially compromises the relationship you have with the patient.

Option D: While withholding analgesia may be inappropriate, reviewing the patient will alert you to their clinical condition and allow you to assess the urgency of the situation.

Option C: This is the least appropriate response. While doctors can refuse to assist in the process leading to and including the procedure of a termination of pregnancy, if the patient experiences complications, they must attend or at least ensure the patient is attended to suitably. This response is also unprofessional as you are ignoring a call for assistance from your nursing colleagues.

Question 46

B, C, E, A, D

Many precautions and safeguards are in place to prevent harm to patients. On occasion these safeguards may fail. The action required at these times must be prioritised. Initially, you must consider the patient – although harm has occurred, it is your duty to limit it and reverse it where possible. Only after this has been completed should you act to inform the patient, before then contributing to the process designed to prevent such incidents from occurring again.

Option B: You must stop the drug immediately. Harm has already been done and you must act to treat the patient. To do this you must remove the underlying cause of harm. Thus, keeping the patient as your primary concern, you must end the ongoing inappropriate treatment first.

Option C: Given that you have stopped the cause of harm, the patient remains your first concern. Assessing the patient will allow you to uncover the extent of the damage done and attempt to treat where possible.

Option E: Informing the sister begins the process of understanding where the system failed with the aim of preventing reoccurrences. Letting the sister know immediately enables her to safeguard other patients and to ensure that they are not also receiving inappropriate drugs.

Option A: Completing an incident form is mandatory at the earliest appropriate time, given that a patient has potentially been exposed to harm. However, it is subordinate to the options above as they pertain directly to patient care and immediate prevention of further harm to others. The incident form is not designed to partition blame, rather it is to understand where the system has failed.

Option D: This is an inappropriate response. It is not proper for you to reprimand a nurse. There is a set process for disciplinary action that involves the nurse's supervisors and it is unprofessional for you to intervene. Furthermore, there is no suggestion that this incident is the fault of the nurse. It is clear that other safeguards have failed, including the doctor who prescribed the inappropriate medication and the pharmacist that failed to spot the error.

Question 47

D, F, G

Team members will occasionally call in sick, and you will be responsible to provide additional cover in their absence. However, this arrangement is normally made on a short-term basis. In this scenario, your colleague with whom you share your workload has informed you that he will be away for a period of time, and is in essence asking that you provide cover for him. When dealing with such situations, you must make an assessment of the episode with a view to ascertaining the amount of time and level of care that you will have to provide. You should consider whether or not your combined actions will present a risk to patient care.

Further to your assessment, you must ensure that the matter is escalated appropriately. Working in a team affords you the support of the other members, including your seniors, and keeping them apprised may help to share the additional workload with an acceptable level of cover. It would be preferred for your colleague to escalate the matter himself, given that escalating on his behalf may compromise his confidentiality.

Option D: Ensuring that the other team members are aware of the situation will work to reduce the burden of his absence upon you. Your SHO may help to take up the slack and reduce your load. This would mean you have more time to spend on individual patients, and would limit the reduction in the quality of care due to being spread thin.

Option F: Your consultant is ultimately responsible for your actions and the care provided by the team. It would be irresponsible to keep the consultant in the dark, as they could arrange alternate solutions to your colleague's absence, potentially including a locum doctor. Not informing the consultant may border on being unprofessional if you are required to lie to them in order to conceal your colleague's absence.

Option G: Talking to your colleague tactfully would allow you to make an adequate assessment of the situation and its implications. If short-term cover for a few hours is required, you may be in a position to facilitate this without compromising care. If a leave of absence for a longer period is required, then it may not be feasible or safe for you to provide this cover and insistence upon senior involvement may be necessary.

Option A: While courtesy dictates that you should allow your colleague the time off, doing so will increase your workload and lead you to the point of exhaustion, causing you to compromise patient care.

Option B: Although this is a good answer, it is superseded by the options listed above. Imposing a reasonable time limit will mean that you provide the necessary cover, but do not compromise yourself and patient care. This response is subordinate to Options D and F, because securing additional support is more conducive to a good work/life balance.

Option C: Advising your colleague to lie is unprofessional for both you and your colleague. This is also not a long-term solution and long-term illness may prompt the employer to request proof.

Option E: While covering for your colleague will preserve your working relationship, it is not a good solution. Covering for long periods of time will compromise patient care and may impact upon your work/life balance. Furthermore, your colleague may not adhere to the necessary number of worked hours to pass her FY1 year.

Option H: Asking your colleague to compensate you for your additional work is insensitive given the personal reasons for his absence. This will negatively affect your working relationship with him.

Question 48

B, D, F

In this scenario, you are faced with a task that must be completed to a deadline. You also have an obligation to your patients to ensure that you deliver safe and optimal care. Staying up to complete the presentation will impact on your ability to perform well the next day. You must therefore decide how best to deal with the demands of your consultant. It is important to maintain your probity and not compromise your professionalism.

Option B: Informing your consultant that you are unable to complete the presentation makes him aware of the dilemma. He may be able to offer additional time to complete the task and you preserve honesty by undertaking this response.

Option D: With patient safety as your top priority, going to sleep ensures you are refreshed and not compromising on patient care by arriving to work tired the next day. Working on the presentation in your spare time ensures that further progress is made ahead of the meeting.

Option F: Providing your consultant with an update ensures that he is aware of what remains to be done in the time you have available before the grand round presentation. Further to Option B, you are providing your consultant with projected time scales so that he may better assess progress.

Option A: This option allows you to complete the presentation at the cost of potentially leaving your team understaffed and compromising patient care. This is both dishonest and unprofessional.

Option C: This is once again unsafe and it may compromise patient care the following day.

Option E: Cancelling the meeting may be appropriate. However, making up an excuse that is untrue is unprofessional and may affect your working relationship with your consultant.

Option G: Asking a colleague may help to complete the presentation in the given time. However, this inconveniences another member of the team, and they may not be well positioned to complete the presentation. They may also have their own responsibilities to attend to, as assigned by the consultant.

Option H: Your consultant may be able to provide guidance on additional content for the presentation and feedback on what you have done already. However, it is not appropriate to ask them to do what you have been assigned, particularly as they are many years your senior and have their own responsibilities to attend to.

Question 49

E, C, A, B, D

Patient safety is an essential theme in this question. Both withholding and administering the medication more frequently are sources of potential harm for the patient. You are therefore risking harm with both actions, and must weigh up which action is most acceptable. Given that the drug is normally administered once-weekly, it is possible that the once-daily dosing is either an off-licence prescription or an error. If you are unable to contact the consultant regarding the management, it is safer to assume that this is indeed a true prescription error. The repercussions of patient harm from an off-licence prescription is less defensible than following the licensed dosages of the drug. As such it is better to under-dose the patient in accordance with the licence than to overdose the patient off-licence under the assumption that this is in keeping with the consultant's intention.

When presented with this scenario, ideally the best course of action would be to refer to the patient's notes to determine the planned management for the patient. The consultant should have documented his intention and the reasons behind an increased dose. If there are any further concerns, another option would be to consult with the hospital pharmacists who may be able to offer further insight or advice on how best to wean the patient off the increased dose.

Option E: Given the options available, getting in touch with the consultant will provide insight into whether the prescription of the increased dose was intentional. This will prevent harm from inappropriate administration or omission of the drug. If this was prescribed in error, the consultant may also be able to provide advice on how best to manage the patient to wean them off the drug.

Option C: If you are unable to access information regarding the veracity of the prescription, the safest response would be to reduce the drug to its licensed dose. This can then be changed in light of further information when the consultant becomes available.

Option A: Leaving the prescription unchanged potentially exposes the patient to an overdose if you are unclear as to whether the increased dose was intentional. However, this is more preferable than causing the patient distress by incorrectly informing them that an error has been made which also impacts on the trust they have in their care providers.

Option B: Speaking to the nurses about any errors your consultant has made does not deal with the situation directly. It fails to deal with the situation at hand, and poorly informs you as to whether this is an instance of a prescription error. Furthermore, the nurses are not in the most appropriate position to determine whether prescribing errors have been made previously. Basing your decision on the views that you elicit are therefore not appropriate.

Option D: Telling the patient that an error has been made is the least appropriate response as you are providing information that may be incorrect and has not yet been established as fact. This may compromise the trust the patient has in your team and impact on their consent for any further interventions. While it is important to inform patients promptly about any errors which are made, unnecessarily causing them distress before confirmation that the incident is indeed an error is not appropriate in this instance.

Question 50

D, C, A, B, E

Acute painful vaso-occlusive crises are a common emergency in patients with sickle cell disease, and require prompt assessment and administration of opiate analgesia. Such patients usually have a care plan, and it is helpful to consult this when treating them. It is useful to obtain a quick history, including a self-assessment of the pain that they are experiencing, any treatments attempted at home, previous hospitalisations and regular medication. Requesting senior advice early is also recommended. Treatment should be commenced without delay, with regular monitoring of pain, and doses modified until pain is controlled. Following acute management, the haematology team at the hospital should be informed at the earliest opportunity.

This particular scenario is further complicated by the patient's background. It is, however, important to remain non-judgemental and treat the patient based on your assessment. Addiction to opioids is a recognised problem in this group of patients, but is less relevant in the acute setting. Consultation with your seniors and the haematology team may help to guide further management, once the acute episode has been addressed with appropriate analgesia, oxygen and fluids.

Option D: Taking a quick history will allow you to elicit further details of the patient's complaint. If the patient is known to the haematological services at the hospital and has a care plan, this will be helpful as it will provide details on how the patient's crises are managed.

Option C: The patient is likely to be well informed about how his crises are managed and the appropriate analgesia that is required to control his pain. While this may be less reliable given this patient's history of drug abuse, the action that results in the least harm in the acute setting is to prescribe the analgesia, rather than allow the patient to continue suffering if this episode is indeed a crisis.

Option A: It is important to investigate any precipitants to the crisis and address these. The patient had been admitted previously with a similar episode; this may be due to drug-seeking behaviour but could be due to an underlying infection that would require treatment with IV antibiotics, once investigation for a source has been undertaken.

Option B: The haematology team will be well informed of patients who are frequently admitted with crises and will have developed care plans for them. A prompt review by the haematology team will aid in the patient's management. However, analgesia should not be withheld until they are reviewed, particularly if there is clinical suspicion that the patient has been admitted with a sickle cell crisis.

Option E: Withholding analgesia when the patient is in pain is the least appropriate response. If there is any doubt, it would be more sensible to prescribe analgesia as a sustaining measure, until the patient is reviewed by a senior member of the team or the haematologists. If this is deemed inappropriate, changes to the patient's management can then be undertaken.

Question 51

D, F, G

This scenario centres around the correct procedures involved in cases where harm has come to a patient, and a complaint is to be made. You must ensure that the patient's intention to complain does not affect your treatment of her but should also ensure that she is aware of the avenues through which she can express her concerns. Further intertwined in this case is the relationship that you have with the nurse and the fact that you must also understand your roles and the boundaries between which you must operate.

It is important to identify that harm has come to a patient given that you have seen that the patient is in pain and that her need for analgesia was neglected. Despite this, you have no evidence that the nurse was truly at fault. It is possible that she was dealing with a more urgent situation and thus unable to attend to this patient. With this in mind, further investigation is clearly required before any disciplinary action is meted out. When answering this question, you may notice that the ideal answers that would be enacted in reality are not options. You must thus choose the most appropriate responses out of less favourable actions.

Option D: Informing the patient of the complaints procedure at their request is part of your duty as a doctor. You are not suggesting that the patient should make a complaint, rather you are informing them of how to do so. A formal complaint will prompt an investigation which will identify any failings in the system and will ensure that the correct remedial action is taken.

Option F: Requesting senior advice may help you to deal with the situation. The scenario is complex and concerns formal action, which may affect your working relationship with colleagues of other professions. Obtaining senior guidance will ensure that the matter is handled sensitively and correctly, and may offer other options that you were not aware of.

Option G: Escalating the complaint to the ward manager is an inappropriate escalation that is selected as a best response, given the subordination of the other options. Completing an incident form in this scenario is mandatory given that harm to a patient has occurred, although this should be one of the last actions to be completed.

Option A: Influencing the patient not to make a complaint would be unprofessional and would cause this incident to be overlooked without investigation. There may be lessons to be learned here, even though nobody may be at fault, and the patient always has a right to complain. The complaint will allow the circumstances to be investigated, and may even clear the nurse of committing an error.

Option B: Reprimanding the nurse is inappropriate. You have no evidence that there was any wrong-doing. Should the nurse be at fault, it is not your role to discipline her and this would thus be unprofessional. There is normally a systematic process in place to deal with events that have the potential to result in patient harm.

Option C: Escalating the complaint to the sister is more appropriate than approaching the ward manager in the first instance. However, completion of an incident form is compulsory and cannot be neglected, since patient harm has occurred.

Option E: Telling the nurse to apologise is akin to Option B, whereby you are disciplining the nurse. This is inappropriate as it falls out of the scope of your role and there is no evidence of wrong-doing.

Option H: Telling the patient, or indeed actually dealing with the complaint, is not advised. There is normally a procedure in place to address complaints and circumventing this by committing yourself to investigate this would be inappropriate.

Question 52

A, E, H

Negotiating with concerned parents must be approached with sensitivity. It can be a very anxious time for parents to attend a GP's surgery seeking medical attention, and their thoughts may not be rationally coordinated. In this scenario, the issue concerns the use of antibiotics in viral illness, which is frequently encountered in clinical practice.

It is a common misconception that antibiotics are a universal therapy and many parents attend surgeries with the hope of obtaining them. It is your duty, however, to address this by re-educating the parent and offering a safety net should they need it, to protect their child as well as yourself. It is important not to fall into inappropriate prescribing due to parental pressure, as this does not justify exposing the child to the potential side-effects of unnecessary medication, and future antibiotic resistance. In these scenarios, the most important remedy is reassurance, while informing the parents that help is available if they remain concerned.

Option A: Exploring the mother's health beliefs may give you an understanding of why she feels there is a need for antibiotics. Uncovering this information will allow you to counter these ideas and more effectively educate the patient by focusing in on specific misconceptions. This will enable you to tailor your advice with greater suitability.

Option E: Providing reassurance and a timeframe for the parent to return is adequate given that your assessment reveals that the patient does not require antibiotics. This response provides a sufficient length of time for the patient to improve before the need to reassess. However, should the condition worsen before that time, the parent is aware that they have the scope to return earlier. This option avoids the prescription of antibiotics, while providing an opportunity for the infant to convalesce naturally.

Option H: This response incorporates another alternative that you can offer in place of antibiotics, which the question has indicated to be unnecessary. Provision of symptomatic treatment may relieve the parent of some of the burden of the child's illness and may also help the child to feed better.

Option B: This would be inappropriate as you are unnecessarily prescribing antibiotics that your clinical assessment has deemed unsuitable. Adversely affecting the mother's confidence is of lesser consequence than potentially harming the child through the side-effects of this medication. This issue can be resolved by justifying your actions and educating the parent.

Option C: This response identifies that the parent's initial presentation may be being used as a ticket of entry to see a doctor for something that is more significant. On this occasion, the child has exhibited signs for the condition that the parent is concerned about and thus it is less likely to be the case. Although this should be explored, it is less suitable in this scenario where more appropriate responses are available, dealing with the complaint at hand.

Option D: It is reasonable to opt to prescribe delayed courses of antibiotics; however, there is a risk that the parent may collect the prescription and administer the medication immediately. This option is superseded by Option E, which offers you the opportunity to reassess before prescribing, which is important particularly if the patient worsens.

Option F: This option is not as appropriate as the answers above as this scenario does not warrant escalation past GP intervention. It is more suitable to inform the parents that they should re-attend at the GP practice in the first instance and should only present to A&E if the situation evolves into an emergency or they require help out of hours.

Option G: Advising the parent that antibiotics are not required is adequate. This response is subordinate to the three selected above as you are not offering an alternative to antibiotics and are not giving the parent any further safety advice. Furthermore, there is no guarantee that the symptoms will completely resolve in the allotted time period, and the parent may no longer remain vigilant to evolving symptoms if given this advice.

Question 53

C, B, A, E, D

As an FY1 on a surgical firm, you have a role to ensure that a constant stream of patients flows through the operating theatres in an efficient manner to minimise the latency periods for the surgeons and anaesthetists. As such, you will need to employ your problem-solving skills to resolve any issues that arise preventing patients from going to theatre.

In this scenario, where a patient has refused to undergo the procedure, his capacity must be questioned. If in the time between him consenting and the time of the surgery, his ability to consent has changed, then he will require further investigation and surgery may not be appropriate. Alternatively, if he has capacity, then you must respect his wishes. In either scenario, you must not neglect to let your seniors know and to seek their advice. If his ability to consent has not been compromised, it would be pertinent to explore the reasons for his refusal and to try to address these as far as you can, to ensure that his procedure takes place.

Option C: Exploring why the patient has suddenly withdrawn consent may uncover a reversible reason which can be dealt with, permitting the patient to have his operation. By conversing with the patient you may also be able to gauge whether his ability to consent has been affected and whether he requires investigation or intervention. This is in keeping with maintaining the patient as your first concern.

Option B: Informing the surgeon and anaesthetists in theatre is important. They will have assessed the patient in the morning and may have further instructions for you to follow, given their knowledge of the patient's case. Since theatre staff have called for the next patient, it is clear that they will be finishing their previous case and should be available to talk to you.

Option A: While you are in discussion with theatre staff, you could liaise with the surgeon and anaesthetist to discuss the possibility of rearranging the theatre list to action the advice they have given you. This will also enable them to optimise the limited theatre time to arrange to call for the next patient rather than waiting on this patient. This option is subordinate to those above, as it is advisable to speak to the patient first to clarify the reasons behind his decision which could be addressed or discussed with your seniors when you get in touch with them.

Option E: This is a reasonable response which is superseded by those above, given that efforts can be made to explore the patient's concerns. If the patient does remain resistant to having the operation despite your efforts, the patient could then be reassured that it will not take place without his agreement. Thus the above actions are more immediate and attempt to promote discussion between ward and theatre staff to optimise the running of the theatre list. Unnecessary delays may prevent other patients from having their surgery if they ultimately run out of theatre time.

Option D: You must respect the patient's right to choose not to have the surgery. A patient cannot be considered unable to make a decision simply because they have made an unwise choice regarding their treatment. This response is therefore the least appropriate option.

Question 54

E, A, D, C, B

Safeguarding children is dependent on effective joint working between agencies and professionals that have different areas of expertise, and also involves working in partnership with parents. Prompt action and appropriate escalation are required here. If there is concern that a child may have been abused or neglected, this should be discussed with a senior colleague and documented in the patient's notes. If these concerns persist following discussion, they should be escalated to the paediatric registrar. If there is evidence that a crime has been committed or that the immediate safety of the child is at risk, the police should also be contacted.

A person may abuse or neglect a child by inflicting harm or by failing to act to prevent harm. The publication 'Working together to safeguard children 2010' reports that: 'All agencies and professionals should be alert to potential indicators of abuse or neglect', and further states that they should 'work co-operatively with parents, unless this is inconsistent with ensuring the child's safety'. Children may be in need of protection in instances where they have suffered harm or are likely to suffer significant harm. Section 47 of the Children Act 1989 gives Children's Social Services a duty to make enquiries to decide whether they must act to safeguard or promote the welfare of the child.

If there are child protection concerns, the patient should not be discharged from hospital without a plan in place to safeguard that child. It is the consultant's responsibility to check that this is in place and the details of this must be recorded in the notes.

Option E: It would be pertinent to establish the facts behind how the injuries were sustained. It is helpful to obtain the mother's account to determine whether it is plausible. If you suspect that the child is being abused, you must act by discussing your concerns with someone more senior.

Option A: Where abuse is suspected, the paediatric registrar must be contacted. This may follow a discussion with a senior colleague.

Option D: This response ensures that your concerns are escalated. However, the options above would be more appropriate. While it may be necessary to contact social services to determine whether the child is known to their service and the reasons why, these actions come after the responses above.

Option C: Confronting the mother will adversely affect your relationship with her, who may react unpredictably to the accusation. If abuse is suspected, the child and family should be advised that there is a need for a review by the paediatric registrar.

Option B: Requesting that the GP follows up your concerns is the least appropriate response. There is a risk that the patient will be lost to follow-up and it exposes the child to harm in the interim. The parent may not attend the appointment with her child, and the record of the patient's GP may be old or inaccurate. It also passes responsibility to another colleague, with an issue that could be dealt with more effectively by the hospital-based team.

Question 55

B, A, E, C, D

Receiving a needle-stick injury can be a stressful situation that must be dealt with promptly and decisively. This is especially the case when dealing with at-risk groups, such as intravenous drug users. There is a clear protocol that should be followed in such an event. The occupational health team is responsible for getting in touch with the patient and arranging for a blood sample to be obtained. This should therefore not be undertaken by the healthcare worker who has sustained the needle-stick injury. Basic measures should be undertaken, which include encouraging the injury to bleed under a tap and seeking help from occupational health during working hours or casualty after hours, for post-exposure prophylaxis.

Option B: When sustaining a needle-stick injury, this action should always be undertaken to minimise the exposure to contaminated blood.

Option A: By reporting to occupational health, you will be able to obtain post-exposure prophylaxis. This will also enable the department to arrange further blood tests for yourself and the patient to determine the risk of contracting a communicable disease.

Option E: While patient harm has not occurred, this is an example of a near miss, for which an incident form must be completed. Despite not being an immediate action, this response supersedes the highly inappropriate responses below.

Option C: Taking blood without consent for the purposes of testing is not in the patient's interest and is unethical. It is noteworthy that the exposed member of staff should not approach the patient themselves, as this will be arranged by occupational health to avoid a conflict of interest.

Option D: Intentionally bleeding into the patient is not only illegal and unethical, but could also expose the patient to harm. It is ranked lower than Option C, due to the greater level of harm caused to the patient. The magnitude of this offence is likely to result in disciplinary action by the GMC.

Question 56

A, E, D, C, B

Articles on new drugs frequently appear in the media. Often the benefits are overstated and reported with a lack of appreciation for the strength of the research. Patients commonly enquire about new drugs and it is the clinician's responsibility to seek the original research paper and review the evidence objectively. It is, however, important not to be cynical and reluctant to incorporate the latest evidence into practice. Patients who present with such articles may do so in the hope that it may relieve the distress that they are experiencing with their condition. This should prompt the clinician to explore the patient's ideas and concerns with a view to providing some solace by offering further measures to help to control their condition.

Option A: Investigating the reasons behind the patient's presentation may uncover concerns regarding his current medication or progression of disease, which should be addressed to provide reassurance and symptomatic relief.

Option E: Acknowledging the patient's request and exploring the available evidence may help to respond to specific questions the patient may have regarding the medication. It is important not to dismiss the patient or the new drug, as this may genuinely have a place in the patient's management. If the evidence for the new drug in this patient's condition is weak, this can then be explained to him with justification as to why it may not be appropriate.

Option D: It is likely that the patient has presented to you as he is dissatisfied with his current level of care regarding his condition. Explaining the reasons behind why you have chosen not to prescribe the new drug and offering alternative measures ensures you are taking active measures to address the issues affecting them.

Option C: This is not ideal as you are not addressing the patient's concerns. You fail to acknowledge the reasons for the patient's presentation or provide adequate justification as to why you are not going to prescribe the drug.

Option B: While it may be inappropriate to prescribe the new drug, using its cost as justification for you not doing so is unlikely to appease the patient. It may seem to the patient that the drug will be effective in his condition but your reluctance is purely driven by its cost. This may have a negative effect on your relationship with the patient, who may seek an unnecessary second opinion or lose trust in the healthcare team.

Question 57

B, E, G

Working as a doctor requires prompt and accurate assessments of situations, including during interactions with patients. With experience, different types of interactions necessitate the employment of different approaches and communication skills. The intention is to promote the patient's trust in both you and the healthcare team by conveying confidence and professionalism. On this basis 'Good Medical Practice' states:

> You must not make malicious and unfounded criticisms of colleagues that may undermine patients' trust in the care or treatment they receive, or in the judgement of those treating them.

Further to the belief that the patient has in her healthcare team, it is important that she does not doubt the quality of care that she has received. As such, questioning reasonable decisions made by previous caregivers should be avoided in the presence of the patient unless serious errors have occurred, about which the patient must be informed.

Option B: Speaking to the patient after the ward round may go some way to repair any damage caused. Explaining or characterising the registrar's comments to be less scathing than initially perceived may reassure the patient that her initial management was not detrimental to her and that your registrar was not in fact undermining the admitting team's decisions.
Option E: Speaking to the registrar after the ward round must be approached sensitively with tact. You should use the interaction to clarify his comments and to broach the topic of undermining colleagues. Speaking to the registrar may enlighten you to the justification for his comments about the admitting team, and this may be relayed to the patient if appropriate. Confrontation is not the best way to approach the registrar, as it will adversely affect your working relationship with him, however, the issue still requires addressing.

Option G: Asking for senior help in addressing this issue is advised. The experience of your SHO may manifest in the quality of advice, and is a middle ground to approaching the registrar directly and escalating the matter to the consultant, both of which have the potential to sour your professional relationship.

Option A: Apologising to the patient for the registrar's comment suggests that the registrar has done something wrong, which may not be the case. He may have justification, which you are unaware of, for the comments that have been made. This apology may also prompt the patient to lose confidence and to question the professionalism in the current medical team prompting her to express reservations about future treatment inappropriately.

Option C: Talking to the admitting team may help you to understand the reasoning behind their decisions. This is, however, of limited use and will not help when talking to your registrar or the patient. Often initial management in the acute setting differs from ongoing care on the wards because of the availability of further information, which better directs specific management.

Option D: Informing the patient of the protocol for making a complaint would be out of context with the situation. The patient has not overtly expressed dissatisfaction at her treatment and has not asked for the procedure involved in making a complaint. Providing this advice in such a manner may provoke an unnecessary complaint against your registrar.

Option F: Speaking to the consultant before speaking to the registrar in question is not preferred in this circumstance. Going immediately above the registrar may damage your working relationship, and is not an appropriate escalation.

Option H: Ignoring the comment does not address the issue. The patient may be losing confidence in the current management and may be questioning your team's professionalism. Furthermore, your registrar may not be aware that his comments were damaging and may need to know to improve his future practice.

Question 58

C, A, D, E, B

Teaching is an important skill to develop in the foundation years. While it is not obligatory to teach students, there is increasing emphasis on taking the time to do so and it is looked upon favourably. With exams approaching, the temptation is for students to spend less time on the wards and more time revising from books. However, spending time on the wards presents potential learning opportunities in areas which are favoured in examinations, particularly practical assessments. It is also worth noting that medical school is the precursor for life as a doctor and, as such, adequate exposure is necessary to assimilate the abilities expected of a foundation doctor.

When a student is attached to a firm, the consultant's responsibility is to ensure that there is adequate exposure to learning opportunities, while the local administrator oversees student attachments.

Option C: The consultant is responsible for the students' education and time on the firm. It would be pertinent to discuss with them any decisions that may affect the teaching agreement the hospital has with the medical school before granting students time off the firm. Your consultant may have arranged a timetable that already accommodates study leave and may have expectations of the students prior to signing them off, upon which you may be impinging.

Option A: This response allows for a compromise, where the students continue to attend but with an agreed plan to address their concerns. Since you are on a busy firm, it is important to note that your ward responsibilities must, however, take priority.

Option D: While it may seem appropriate to suggest that the students join another FY1, this may actually go against the wishes of your consultant, and indeed those of the team you have suggested that they join. Your consultant may again have issues with sign-off at the end of their placement and you are passing responsibility to a colleague, who will have their own responsibilities to attend to. Therefore such arrangements must be cleared with your colleague's team as well as with your own. This response is, however, preferred to Option E, as it does attempt to address the students' concerns, and may be accepted if it is agreed by both teams.

Option E: Insisting that the students continue to attend is less appropriate as it fails to address their concerns. They have highlighted their intention to take time off to revise, and you are not acting to acknowledge or accommodate this.

Option B: This is the least appropriate response, as you do not have sufficient authority to grant them time off. This may go against both the consultant's and the medical school's wishes, and you may have to explain yourself to them if this issue is raised.

Question 59

A, F, G

On occasion, healthcare professionals may disagree on a patient's management. Nurses are responsible for attending to the daily needs of the patient and may therefore be more informed about a patient's complaint. In this scenario, the nurse may have more information that is pertinent to the patient's pain management which may explain her reluctance to follow your plan. Ensuring patient safety is important and it is therefore necessary to explore the nurse's views and review the patient's case to ensure that you have not missed anything.

Option A: It would be sensible to discuss the case with a senior colleague if there is a difference of opinion regarding the best management for the patient. This may shed light on important factors that need to be considered for this patient.

Option F: Reviewing the patient again may uncover important factors that had been overlooked the first time. This may help to determine the most appropriate management of the patient's complaint.

Option G: You are on-call and this is not one of your regular patients. The nurse may therefore be more informed about the patient's case. Discussing her reservations may uncover something that you may have missed when you first reviewed the patient.

Option B: This response would affect your working relationship with your colleague and fails to explore the reasons behind her actions.

Option C: Before a decision is reached regarding the suitability of what you have prescribed, you must explore the nurse's views. It may be that what you have prescribed is indeed appropriate and this comes from reviewing the patient and their complaint thoroughly. Your decision should be complemented by the nurse's input as opposed to instinctively overruled.

Option D: It may be appropriate to discuss the incident privately once the episode is over. However, this response is superseded by Option G, as it fails to address the problem directly and does not concentrate on whether the patient truly needs analgesia.

Option E: While it may be necessary to document what has happened, this response fails to address the problem. The patient is in pain and discussing the case with your colleagues and reviewing the patient again take precedence.

Option H: It is necessary to respect the contribution of your colleagues and as such you should acknowledge the reasons behind the nurse's decision. Insisting that she gives the medication fails to address this, and could potentially put the patient at risk, if it evolves that the patient does not require further analgesia.

Question 60

C, D, E, B, A

As a foundation trainee, you will frequently encounter pressure from other members of the healthcare team, seeking to use their influence in completing the tasks associated with their roles. On occasion, these tasks or objectives may conflict with your own. Your responsibility is to ensure patient safety is not compromised and that you attend to jobs of the highest priority first.

As an FY1, you should avoid making decisions to discharge patients. This should be deferred to more senior colleagues. You are, however, responsible for your actions in an inappropriate discharge. In this scenario, you must determine whether or not it would be safe to discharge this patient, given the new information that has become available. The original decision that was made by your consultant in the morning would need to be reassessed in light of the blood results. Since the patient is immunocompromised with recent chemotherapy and demonstrates signs of a brewing infection, it would be irresponsible to discharge them without senior review. With patient safety as your primary concern, you should not allow yourself to be coerced into sending the patient home in order to appease the bed manager.

Option C: Discussing the case with a more experienced colleague would help clarify your concerns and ensure that the patient is reviewed ahead of potential discharge. This response is preferred to Option D as it allows for a definitive decision at an earlier opportunity, providing the patient and your colleagues with a clearer idea as to whether he will be discharged or kept in for overnight observation.

Option D: Erring on the side of caution and postponing discharge would cause least harm to the patient, particularly if you are concerned. This provides further opportunity for the patient to be reviewed by a more senior colleague, if one is not immediately available. This patient is at risk of sepsis which may be clinically silent but equally devastating; discharging him when there is concern may be detrimental. Overnight observation of the patient ensures that early signs of deterioration are picked up and acted upon.

Option E: Discussing the situation with the patient is not as safe as definitively keeping the patient in hospital overnight. It does, however, leave scope to retain the patient, as opposed to the following responses in which the patient is discharged and exposed to the greatest risk of harm.

Option B: Allowing the patient to go home without a senior review is inappropriate, as the risk to the patient has been identified. Arranging for the patient to be followed up in two weeks is not an appropriate safety net, as his deterioration is likely to be far more rapid. This response is, however, favoured to a discharge with no scheduled follow-up.

Option A: This is the most inappropriate option, as the patient has been discharged with no follow-up arranged.

Question 61

C, E, A, B, D

Medical certificates, including those associated with death, should be completed to the best of your ability with information that you hold to be true. Dishonestly completing forms and documents with false information goes against GMC guidance on probity published in 'Good Medical Practice', which states:

You must do your best to make sure that any documents are not false or misleading. This means that you must take reasonable steps to verify the information in the documents, and that you must not deliberately leave out relevant information.

Given that you do not agree with the consultant's decision, it is clear that you do not feel that bronchopneumonia is responsible, and thus publishing that it is would in fact be dishonest. As your consultant is not available, generally speaking, it would not be advisable to complete the certificate as it would involve providing information you do not accept.

Option C: Obtaining further advice from a senior is advisable. Your registrar may be able to explain the consultant's decision and highlight important points that you may have overlooked. Alternatively, the registrar may opt to complete the certificate themselves, or side with you and may endorse an alternative cause of death. The joint decision and its justification can then be relayed to the consultant, who would be assured that you did not oppose the decision without consulting others.

Option E: The coroner's representatives are always available to offer advice and support. Explaining the circumstances and facts surrounding the death would help them to ascertain whether bronchopneumonia is reasonable as a cause of death. Having had the discussion, there is not an obligation to complete the certificate if you remain uncomfortable with the agreed cause of death.

Option A: Completing the form with an acceptable cause of death which you sincerely believe to be the case is preferred over the options below. It may affect your relationship with the consultant as you did not discuss this further, but it is better than not completing the form which is insensitive to the deceased's family.

Option B: Not completing the form prevents the family from proceeding with funeral arrangements. While this is not ideal, it is preferable to providing false information and this response may present an opportunity for someone else to complete the form. This option may also affect your professional relationship with the consultant, as you have not followed their instructions.

Option D: Obeying your consultant's orders when you believe the cause of death to be incorrect goes against good practice. It is essentially dishonest and, while this action may please your consultant, it will contribute to skewing national statistics on causes of death, which then affect the health areas upon which the government divides funds.

Question 62

C, G, H

There are several issues that must be dealt with in this scenario. Your first priority is the patient and to ensure that they are stable and have not suffered any adverse reactions due to the expired vaccine. Your professional integrity is important here, and there is a need to be open and honest about what has happened. You are accountable for the mistake that was made, as it is necessary to check the details of any drug or vaccine, including its expiry date before it is given to a patient. When things do go wrong, the GMC publication 'Good Medical Practice' states that:

> *… you must act immediately to put matters right, if that is possible. You should offer an apology and explain fully and promptly to the patient what has happened, and the likely short-term and long-term effects.*

The second issue to deal with is the nurse's reaction to the error. This is of lower importance than ensuring that the patient's well-being is not compromised. Discussing the issue with the nurse would be appropriate. An incident form must also be completed since a patient has potentially come to harm.

Option C: It would be appropriate to get in touch with the parents to ensure that the patient is not suffering from any adverse effects. In accordance with GMC guidance, a full explanation must be offered, together with a plan to remedy the situation. If the patient is compromised from administration of the expired vaccine, arrangements should be made for readmission.

Option G: Resolving the issue with the nurse is of lower priority, but having a discussion with her about what has happened and completion of an incident form is necessary. This is more appropriate than other options which avoid completing the incident form, since the event should be investigated and measures put in place to prevent future recurrence.

Option H: This response is not ideal, but more appropriate than the other options which are available. It would be sensible to seek senior advice. Seeking the advice of a senior colleague, while not a member of your team, may help to prioritise your actions. All members of the healthcare team will share the understanding that patient safety is the top concern, as per GMC guidance.

Option A: Escalating the issue to the ward sister may be necessary. However, placing blame on the nurse and complaining about her lack of professionalism will negatively affect your working relationship with her. It would be more appropriate to have an open and frank discussion about what has occurred with a view to resolving the issue and preventing recurrence.

Option B: While it would be appropriate to contact the parents and explain what has happened, you should not provide reassurance on something you cannot guarantee. Providing the parents with the option of returning if they had any concerns allows for a plan to be put in place in the event of any adverse effects.

Option D: Contacting the parents would be appropriate, but a full and honest explanation must be offered. While this may cause distress, it would cause less harm than withholding information which may be perceived negatively by the patient's family, and the resultant effect it would have on your relationship with them.

Option E: It would be necessary to discuss the incident with the nurse who was involved. However, an incident form must be completed to ensure measures are put in place to avoid recurrence.

Option F: This would not be appropriate as it does not address the issue and negatively impacts on your working relationship with the nurse.

Question 63

D, B, A, E, C

Patients with capacity are permitted to change their mind about whether to proceed with surgery, regardless of how late this decision is made. It is advisable to explore the reasons behind their decision, since issues can sometimes be resolved or a compromise can be found. If a patient is concerned about potential side-effects post-surgery, reassurance can be provided. If their decision relates to practical issues, potential solutions can be offered. If this does not resolve the issue and patients wish to be discharged, this should be permitted provided that they know the potential implications to their health or well-being by doing so.

Option D: It would be appropriate to explain the potential risks of leaving, in order to ensure the patient is aware of these should he wish to leave without surgery. The patient is then able to make an informed decision about his care.

Option B: The patient should be permitted to leave if he wishes to do so. It may be possible for the patient to still undergo surgery if he returns promptly before the end of the list.

Option A: The patient's family are aware of his admission. It is therefore possible to get in touch with his wife without breaching confidentiality. This response may help to persuade the patient to remain in hospital and a compromise to be reached regarding the reasons why he must leave.

Option E: This response is not ideal as it passes responsibility for his care to another colleague. However, it ensures the patient is followed up in the community to monitor his condition and reassess whether he would still need surgery.

Option C: This is the least appropriate response, as the patient has capacity and should be allowed to leave if he wishes to do so. The patient is able to weigh his options and is fully aware of the implications of not having the surgery so it would be inappropriate to forcibly keep him in hospital.

Question 64

A, D, B, C, E

You will frequently encounter patients who have misconceptions about medical care and treatment options. It is your responsibility to present the evidence to the patient that allows them to make an informed decision. It is important here that your personal views do not feature in the information you provide patients. The GMC states:

> You must not express to your patients your personal beliefs, including ... moral beliefs, in ways that exploit their vulnerability or that are likely to cause them distress.

It is, however, acceptable to provide medical advice based on your professional opinion.

This scenario is complicated by a mother who has made a decision on behalf of her child. This right is afforded to a parent provided that they have all the information they need to make an informed decision. This is a complex area that raises questions regarding the rights of a child to protection from ill health versus the rights of a parent to make choices for their child.

'The United Nations Convention on the Rights of the Child' contains a comprehensive list that includes a child's right to 'the highest attainable standard of health' and includes access to 'preventative healthcare' (Article 24). However, also contained in the treaty is the duty of governments to 'respect the responsibilities, rights and duties of parents or guardians ... to provide ... appropriate direction and guidance' (Articles 5, 14). In addition, the British Medical Association (BMA) states that 'parents have the right to be involved in important decisions concerning their children' (BMA Guidance, 2003).

In the UK, childhood vaccination is not compulsory, although levels of immunisation are high. The relatively low risk of contracting most of the infectious diseases which are routinely immunised against in the UK means that compelling parents to immunise their children is not justified. In addition, compulsory immunisation does not guarantee universal uptake. Education and support is therefore more likely to lead to positive outcomes.

Option A: Your first priority must be the well-being of the patient, so it would be appropriate to ensure that she is stable.

Option D: Exploring the reasons behind the parent's decision not to immunise her child may uncover her reasons for not doing so. It is the parent's choice whether her child is immunised or not.

Option B: The parent may be unaware of the risks of not immunising her child. Her misconceptions could be addressed with education regarding the benefits of immunisation, which may reduce the risks to her child in the future.

Option C: There is no guarantee that the child's presentation is due to her not being immunised. As stated above, you should not express your personal views in the treatment of patients in a manner that would cause them undue harm.

Option E: Refusing to treat the patient is the least appropriate response. The child requires medical attention and she should be your first priority. You should also not let your personal views affect your treatment of patients.

Question 65

B, F, G

Patients may disagree with the recommended medical advice regarding their management. It is important that the ultimate management plans hinge on the patient's preferences and willingness to submit to the recommended treatment. When a patient refuses to consent to a treatment, their capacity should be questioned as appropriate, in accordance with the Mental Capacity Act 2005. This states that patients must be able to understand the relevant information, retain, weigh and communicate that decision. Importantly, a patient cannot be considered unable to make a decision because they have made an unwise choice regarding their treatment.

In this scenario, there is no suggestion that the patient has diminished capacity and if, after ensuring that she is aware of the risks of her decision, she still refuses treatment, you must respect her decision. Thus, you must ensure that you have given the patient all the information that she requires and that she is aware of the advantages and disadvantages of all the options. If possible, you should endeavour to address any issues or obstacles that are preventing the patient from considering her option.

Option B: Ensuring that the patient is aware of all the options available to her is essential for her to reach a decision on how she wishes to proceed. It is important that she is aware of the risks of refusing surgery, the intervention your team has deemed to be the most suitable option for her.

Option F: Eliciting further information about her plans for alternative therapies will allow you to research these and find out their efficacy in this condition. Armed with the relevant evidenced-based knowledge will better prepare you to answer her questions and present the available options and their realistic value.

Option G: It would be necessary to determine her reasons for refusing surgery so that these can be addressed where possible. The patient may have misconceptions about the treatment options which can be dispelled. This response would also build rapport, and the patient will appreciate your efforts in promoting a shared decision-making process.

Option A: There is no reason to doubt the patient's ability to make decisions and so there are no grounds to act in the patient's best interests. Taking blood for the purposes of surgery breaches the patient's trust in you as her treating clinician and will adversely affect the doctor–patient relationship.

Option C: While it may be true that refusing surgery puts the patient's life at risk, there are more appropriate responses available for dealing with this scenario. It is, however, important to make the patient aware of this risk, so that she understands the implications of her decision. It would be advisable to have all the relevant information regarding the alternative therapies and their evidence base, before conveying that surgery is most likely to prolong life. It is worth noting, however, that surgery in this case offers the best chance for curative therapy, while medical therapies are unlikely to have the same impact on her condition.

Option D: There is no evidence to suggest that the patient is suffering from an acute confusional state. The Mental Capacity Act 2005 states that 'a person must be assumed to have capacity unless it is established that he lacks capacity'. With the absence of evidence to suggest that the patient lacks capacity, it must be assumed.

Option E: This is inappropriate as you cannot substantiate the statement. It is important that you do not dismiss alternative medicine and promote Western methods as being more effective without evidence.

Option H: Contacting a relative with reference to specific management would breach the patient's right to confidentiality. Before contacting a relative you must get consent from the patient.

Question 66

D, C, B, A, E

Patients may frequently attend following poor compliance to your recommended treatment. The patient has the right to autonomy, and provided that she is fully informed about their condition and the impact of her choices, you should respect her decisions. You must, however, take every opportunity to educate her and ensure that she is fully aware of the consequences of not following the recommended advice. Further discussion may also shed light on the reasons for poor adherence, which could be addressed through exploration of alternative measures and reinforced with medical literature. In support, the GMC states:

> You should encourage patients ... to take an interest in their health and to take action to improve and maintain it. This may include advising patients on the effects of their life choices on their health and well-being and the possible outcomes of their treatments.

It would also be sensible to arrange a follow-up appointment to monitor progress. If a patient with full capacity continues to refuse, you must respect this decision. You should continue to act in the patient's best interest and offer any treatments the patient may be amenable to, including appropriate follow-up.

Option D: Your first concern should be treating the patient and ensuring that she is stabilised. Other responses are subordinate to ensuring that the patient is safe.

Option C: You have a duty of beneficence to ensure that the patient is fully aware of the risk she exposes herself to through poor compliance. Despite previous admissions, you should make every effort to explore her current level of knowledge and provide education on the impact of her current level of care.

Option B: Providing the patient with literature helps to reinforce the information you have provided and summarises important aspects of what you have said. This also allows for the patient to review the information again which may help to improve her current level of adherence to treatment.

Option A: While it is important to stabilise the patient, dismissing the value of patient education would not be appropriate. You must act in the patient's best interests and ensure that she is fully aware of the implications of her actions. This may also help to empower her to take responsibility for the control of her condition.

Option E: This is the least appropriate response, as it breaches the patient's confidentiality. It also removes responsibility from the patient. As stated by the GMC above, you should promote self-care wherever possible.

Question 67

D, B, E, C, A

Some travel vaccinations are available on the NHS while others must be paid for. This can sometimes lead to an expensive bill for a number of vaccinations. It is the patient's choice as to whether or not they opt for these injections, as there is no restriction on travel without vaccinations.

In these scenarios, the patient should always be afforded all the information available including the risks he is taking by not having the immunisations, and the effects of the diseases. In doing this, the patient will be making a fully informed decision, and the conversation itself should be documented. In place of vaccinations, it would be pertinent to supply the patient with alternative information on disease prevention.

Option D: Providing advice is free and acts as a safety net given that he has declined vaccinations. This will protect the patient against a myriad of diseases including those for which he has not been vaccinated against as well as other common diseases. Advice is superior to chemical prophylaxis, given that there are no side-effects and that a broader range of diseases are guarded against.

Option B: Supplying chemical prophylaxis may be cheaper than vaccinations and be more amenable to the patient. It will protect him against a smaller range of diseases and is unlikely to cover him for the vaccinations that he has refused. Using medication for these purposes still exposes the patient to the potential side-effects of such drugs; however, this is outweighed by the risk of harm from actually contracting the disease.

Option E: Informing the patient of the warning signs of diseases allows for early disease recognition enabling the patient to seek medical attention, and acts as a further safety net. In general, prophylaxis is preferred to this type of advice as it protects against the harm caused by contracting a disease.

Option C: Allowing the patient to leave would not be appropriate as you need to ensure that he is fully aware of the consequences of his actions.

Despite his refusal of the immunisations, he should still be afforded further advice on other measures he can take to protect himself.

Option A: This option is the least appropriate, as it is dishonest to defraud the NHS by providing vaccinations which are not covered. This is both unprofessional and goes against GMC guidance on probity.

Question 68

A, E, C, D, B

Protecting vulnerable adults and dealing with abuse can be challenging. A vulnerable adult is defined as: 'A person aged 18 or over who is or may be in need of community care services by reason of mental or other disability, age or illness; who is or may be unable to protect him or herself against significant harm or exploitation' (Law Commission, 1997). Abuse may be physical, psychological, sexual, financial or discriminatory, and includes neglect and acts of omission. Ignoring the medical or physical care needs of a patient or withholding the necessities of life including medication or adequate nutrition also constitute abuse.

As in this scenario, if you believe a patient is being abused and that they lack capacity to consent to disclosure, you must give the information to an appropriate responsible person or authority. GMC guidance in the publication 'Confidentiality' states that this is acceptable, since you believe the disclosure is in the patient's best interests and necessary to protect others from risk of serious harm. The patient is from a nursing home, and it is possible that others residing in the same institution may be suffering from abuse or neglect. It is therefore imperative that you take the necessary action to ensure that these concerns are adequately assessed and investigated.

Option A: Taking a history from the patient, wherever possible, or a collateral history would be appropriate to establish the facts. This would give further information regarding the circumstances leading to admission. As stated above, if abuse is suspected these concerns should be relayed to someone more senior, such as your registrar or consultant who will investigate further. An initial exploration may help you to rule out abuse and prevent you from escalating an innocuous matter unnecessarily.

Option E: In serious issues, such as safeguarding, you must always inform a senior precluding further formal action. Their experience and sanction are important and may prevent an inappropriate escalation, where you may be the source of a serious allegation that turns out to be unfounded. A senior colleague will be able to evaluate the necessary information, including mental capacity, consent, medical attention and the need for urgent action.

Option C: You must treat all cases of potential abuse seriously, and take any immediate steps that are practical to ensure the safety of the abused person. Your senior colleague will determine what action should be taken, and can make a referral to a social worker, who will establish the level of risk and proceed with investigations.

Option D: Requesting that the GP follows up your concerns would be inappropriate. Passing responsibility to another health professional will lead to delays and the loss of information in handover, with the patient exposed to potential harm in the interim. All members of staff have a responsibility to act on concerns of abuse and action must therefore be taken promptly.

Option B: Not taking any action is clearly the least appropriate response. You must act on your concerns, and inform the relevant people that abuse may have occurred.

Question 69

C, G, H

You will frequently share your clinical experiences with colleagues, and this provides an opportunity to reflect and improve. When you or your colleagues experience difficulties, it can be helpful to share these with colleagues who may be in a position to offer help and advice. When a more senior colleague confides in you, similar principles apply but the advice you are able to offer may be more limited given your relative inexperience. The work of a more senior colleague differs in that it is more demanding and carries greater responsibility. Therefore any problems may have to be dealt with slightly differently, by approaching doctors of the same grade or more senior.

Option C: Suggesting that your registrar speaks to colleagues of a similar grade may be beneficial. Her peers may be more suited to offering advice on how to manage the increased demands of her new job. Some may have been in a similar position and may be able to speak from experience.

Option G: Spending time exploring the difficulties that your registrar is having may offer a clearer insight into the situation and is likely to be therapeutic in its own right. The issues that arise may be amenable to solutions which may ease the difficulties she is currently experiencing.

Option H: Suggesting that your registrar speaks to your consultant is beneficial as it directly addresses the issue. An assessment must also be made here as to whether patient safety is being put at risk, and the necessary measures to deal with this put in place. While it may offer your registrar some comfort, there is no real need for you to be present during this meeting and it may be more beneficial if it were a private discussion. This response is, however, more suitable than the other options which are available.

Option A: Your registrar's work is likely to be more complex and you are unlikely to be able to provide much assistance. This option also fails to resolve the issue and is not a long-term solution to the problem that the registrar has highlighted.

Option B: Your registrar has only just come back from a period of absence and this may partly explain the difficulties she is having integrating back into her clinical responsibilities. This response merely avoids the problem rather than directly addressing it. This will also result in recurrence of the problem when the registrar needs to return to work after this additional time off.

Option D: The registrar may benefit from counselling, though this may not be available instantly. Other responses are available which directly address the issue and are more immediate.

Option E: Your registrar will have a greater idea about her principal challenges and is therefore best suited to having the discussion with the consultant. Also, approaching your consultant without the registrar's consent or knowledge may adversely affect your working relationship with her.

Option F: Asking other members of the team to be more supportive is not a long-term solution and removes the responsibility of dealing with the problem from your registrar. It also publicises the problem that she has confided in you, which she may not appreciate.

Question 70

E, B, A, C, D

This presents a difficult scenario to deal with, having to balance the courtesy you must show your colleagues with your duty to protect patients. The fact that there is a half-empty bottle of wine and the effects this has had on your colleague's appearance provide reasonable grounds to conclude that he is drinking while on duty. It is important, however, to remain non-confrontational and avoid incriminating your colleague; there may be reasons to explain his actions and you should remain supportive.

In instances where the evidence is less conclusive, you should determine the facts before reaching conclusions or unfairly judging your colleagues. In this scenario, there is a potential risk to patient care and so you must not ignore what you have seen.

Option E: Speaking to your colleague will allow you to elicit further details about what you have seen. It may also uncover the reasons behind his actions, which will permit you to offer support as necessary. This also provides an opening to sensitively explain that he should not be working in his current condition, and in this manner take direct action to prevent harm to patients.

Option B: Speaking to your consultant is the next appropriate option. It is important that you do not ignore what you have seen; if patients are being put at risk, you must act.

Option A: This response escalates the issue excessively and will adversely affect your working relationship with your colleague. It is, however, preferred to the options below, as it ensures that the problem is addressed in order to protect patients.

Option C: Discussing the issue with other FY1s would unnecessarily delay your actions and will put patients at risk in the interim. They are also unlikely to be able to offer you advice that will significantly help with the situation. If your colleague is experiencing problems, publicising this would exacerbate the problems and will be detrimental to your working relationship.

Option D: You must not ignore what you have seen, since patients are potentially at risk. You should therefore take steps to address the issue by protecting patients, and ensuring that your colleague receives the support he needs.

Question 71

B, C, F

As a foundation trainee, you are required to continue developing the skills you learnt at medical school. This includes taking responsibility for your own learning by arranging supervised learning events with your seniors. You must demonstrate your willingness to learn from others and be open to and accepting of feedback from your colleagues. In this scenario, you have an uncomfortable experience with your clinical supervisor who has agreed to supervise you. While there will be instances where your shortcomings are exposed, it is important to learn from these and recognise the constructive feedback you receive as being essential for your professional development.

Option B: Discussing your experience with the clinical supervisor will allow you to determine areas that need further improvement, as you will receive constructive feedback on your performance. Your own view of what happened during the assessment may differ from that of the supervisor so it would be helpful to discuss this with him. In addition, the supervisor may appreciate how you felt during the assessment and decide to alter the structure of the learning event in future to permit further questioning once you have left the patient's bedside.

Option C: As you feel quite strongly about the uncomfortable position you were placed in during the assessment, it would be sensible to allow some time to compose yourself and plan what you wish to discuss before speaking to your supervisor. It is important not to come across as confrontational, as this will harm your working relationship with the consultant and impact on further assessments that you require him to complete.

Option F: It is important to reflect on your experiences in order to learn from previous encounters. This will enable you to improve on the next assessment. Your supervisor will appreciate that you have learnt from your mistakes and listened to his advice.

Option A: While you may have felt embarrassed by your supervisor's actions, it is not clear that he is at fault. Escalating the issue to the programme director before discussing the matter with your supervisor will adversely affect your working relationship with him. It would also potentially compromise any further learning events requests you have for him.

Option D: The clinical supervisor is not responsible for any wrong-doing in relation to the patient or their care and an apology would therefore be unnecessary.

Option E: This response fails to address the issue. You may continue to have negative feelings about the experience and towards your supervisor, which is likely to affect your working relationship with him and the future assessments you may require him to do.

Option G: While it may help you to discuss your experience with your colleagues, this response fails to directly resolve the issue. You may have misinterpreted the supervisor's actions and it would be more beneficial to discuss these with him.

Option H: It is important that you display an eagerness to learn and remain open towards varied teaching styles. Acknowledging your errors from this assessment and acting on the constructive feedback that you receive will allow you to improve at the next assessment you do with this consultant.

Question 72

C, D, E, B, A

When personal friendships and relationships interact with professional life, various dilemmas can arise. Separating the personal aspects from your professional management of a patient, with whom you are close, can be very difficult and may affect the relationship in question. Furthermore, clinical judgement and assessment in these circumstances can ultimately be clouded and biased by the nature of the personal relationship. These concerns have led to guidance in the publication 'Good Medical Practice' to state that 'wherever possible, you should avoid providing medical care to anyone with whom you have a close personal relationship'.

While this scenario is slightly removed from this guidance as you are not treating your friend's mother, some of the principles still apply. Your close relationship with your friend may cause you to act in a manner that may compromise your integrity and the patient's confidentiality. Given that you do not belong to the team looking after the patient, you should not attempt to obtain confidential data belonging to the patient. Doing so will bring your probity and integrity into question and may even go as far as bringing the profession into disrepute. When resolving this scenario, it is important that you act in a manner becoming of a doctor, while respecting the confidentiality of your friend's mother, and maintaining a positive relationship with your friend.

Option C: Speaking to the consultant responsible for care may appear drastic, but it is a measure that isolates you from this scenario. The consultant will be aware that communication is required with the patient's son, and simultaneously you will not have violated the patient's confidentiality while ensuring that your friend is kept updated.

Option D: Asking for the patient's consent to update your friend will ensure that you have not inappropriately broken the patient's confidentiality. This option is subordinate to Option C because it involves your direct input and assessment of the patient's clinical care, which is ill advised given your closeness to this case.

Option E: Explaining that Trust policy forbids you from intervening will protect you from breaking the patient's confidentiality and compromising your integrity. This response may, however, affect your friendship, but it is preferred to the responses below, given that you are explaining the formal reason for not obtaining the information required by your friend.

Option B: Refusing to provide any information will again prevent any inappropriate compromise of confidentiality and your integrity, but is more likely to negatively affect your friendship than Option E and is thus ranked lower.

Option A: Obtaining the information and passing it on to your friend is a serious breach of GMC guidance, specifically on the subject of confidentiality and probity. The patient may wish for her medical records to remain confidential, and you must not assume that the intimacy of her relationship allows for disclosures to be made without consent.

Question 73

D, B, E, C, A

Completing the e-Portfolio is an important part of your FY1 year, and is required in order to be signed off at the end and allow progression to FY2. As such, it should not be neglected and should be updated regularly. The skills that must be demonstrated, for which evidence must be provided, are procedures that are performed on a regular basis and are tested as part of your development as a doctor. They are commonly performed in a normal working day and should not require additional time or special arrangements to undertake.

In the process of completing the tasks associated with the e-Portfolio, you must remember that your patients should always be your first priority, and safety should not be compromised in any way in order to complete the targets and supervised learning events. Just as probity and integrity are important in your conduct with patients, they are also important with other members of staff such as your educational supervisor.

Option D: Meeting your supervisor on time is preferred, given that organisation and punctuality are important attributes expected in a doctor. It may be understandable why you have not completed your targets to date and offering another meeting in two weeks to reassess your progress demonstrates dedication and flexibility in order to achieve them.

Option B: Explaining to your supervisor why the assessments are incomplete will help them to recognise that you require input and guidance, but are willing to achieve your goals. This response is subordinate to Option D, only in that you are not offering a solution to the current predicament.

Option E: Staying back later to complete your targets and practical skills demonstrates dedication but is also an example of being unable to maintain your work/life balance. The e-Portfolio should be updated through the course of the year and so staying late after work is not a sustainable response. The supervised learning events are intended to be completed during the working day and you should not have to stay back to fulfil them. This response is preferred to those below, however, given that you are preserving honesty and integrity in this approach.

Option C: Changing targets on your e-Portfolio is not advisable. Targets are tailored to your own personal development and should not be changed in order to be less demanding, as this is not honest or conducive to your progress. Furthermore, duping your supervisor is unprofessional and discourteous.

Option A: Manipulating the situation in an attempt to avoid your supervisor is unprofessional, dishonest and unbecoming of a doctor. Meeting educational supervisors later than prescribed on your e-Portfolio demonstrates a lack of organisation, and may require an explanation in the future.

Question 74

A, C, F

While no specific dress code exists for doctors, you must ensure that you dress in a way that maintains trust in the profession. Not doing so may compromise the relationship you have with patients. Medical students are on a vocational course that prepares them ultimately to practise as doctors, and therefore these rules are extrapolated to include them as well. In this scenario, a senior colleague has flagged up what he feels is the inappropriate attire of a student. You must take the issue seriously and take measures to correct this, especially since this could be a precursor to a patient making a complaint about the issue.

Option A: Having an informal discussion with the student allows for the issue to be addressed without senior involvement. This avoids any undue embarrassment that may be caused by involving more senior figures in the event a complaint is made by a patient or the consultant is made aware. Sensitively explaining the situation privately gives the student the opportunity to resolve the issue.

Option C: Of the responses which are available, asking a senior to talk to the student may be appropriate. He may be sufficiently removed from the situation and have the authority to have a discussion with her without significantly impacting on their working relationship. This option is not ideal in that you are likely to be in most contact with the student during the day, and it passes responsibility to another colleague.

Option F: The local administrators at the hospital are responsible for student issues regarding their clinical placement. They may be more appropriately positioned to have this discussion with the student, which can ensure that it does not affect the working relationship with any specific team member. They also have sufficient authority to raise the issue with the student.

Option B: The registrar from the other team has raised the issue so it would be prudent to take the matter seriously. It may adversely affect your relationship with him if you fail to act and the student continues to dress inappropriately. If a patient were to complain about the student's dress code, the issue may have to be escalated to more senior figures and this would cause undue embarrassment, which could be avoided if it is addressed before it gets to that stage.

Option D: Involving more colleagues may help in guiding how best to approach the issue. This, however, may cause unnecessary delays and publicises the issue so that more people are aware of it. This may make the student uncomfortable, particularly if more of your colleagues are discussing the issue. If this were to get back to her, it may be misinterpreted as gossip and adversely affect the working relationship you have with her.

Option E: While this response attempts to deal with the issue, it is unlikely to have the desired effect. Specifying the problem will enable her to make a more sound judgement in the future regarding her attire. This approach may be prompted by your desire not to cause offence, but an open and frank discussion is more likely to resolve the issue. This response may also be interpreted as a personal opinion rather than what a senior colleague has asked you to address.

Option G: The registrar has approached you regarding the issue as he feels that you are more suited to having this discussion with the student. Requesting that he addresses the issue himself removes the responsibility from you, and he is unlikely to appreciate your decision given that he has approached you for help.

Option H: The registrar has approached you as he feels there is a problem. Addressing the problem would avoid further issues that may arise in the future if a patient were to complain or a consultant flags the issue.

Question 75

D, E, F

Most hospitals incorporate the on-call FY1 into the crash team. This places you among the first responders in a hospital emergency. On most occasions during the day, and when in attendance in A&E, you are likely to find that you are the second wave to arrive, and that CPR has begun under the supervision of a senior doctor. In these circumstances, it is important to slot in and be proactive in completing whatever needs to be done, be it taking an arterial blood gas (ABG) sample or performing chest compressions.

When providing ward cover, however, you may find that you are the first doctor on the scene, and thus must take charge of the scenario. In a crash call, you should liaise with other health professionals on the ward who may know the patient, and can advise on whether they are for resuscitation or not. Usually when a cardiac arrest call is made, this is because the patient is for resuscitation, however, you must be wary that errors can be made.

Advanced life support (ALS) should be started immediately and the patient's desire for resuscitation should be assumed, unless a valid DNAR form is found. If a form is present, CPR must be stopped immediately. It is important to note that a DNAR form is an order against CPR, but not active treatment if the patient shows signs of life. Thus, the next step after terminating CPR should be to search for signs of life and adopt the ABCDE approach if signs persist.

Option D: Given that a DNAR order has been found, CPR should cease. Opening the airway will further assist in assessing the patient's breathing as a sign of life.

Option E: After CPR has stopped, the patient needs to be assessed for life in order to decide the next action. Should the patient be breathing and their heart beating, then the ABCDE approach should be used to support the patient.

Option F: This response further checks the patient for signs of life in addition to Option E in order to assess suitability for further management.

Option A: Taking a blood gas sample is not currently appropriate. Blood gases may be taken as part of ALS, however, ALS should not be instituted in this case. Should the patient show signs of life after stopping CPR, then it would be acceptable to perform an ABG as part of the 'Breathing' stage of the ABCDE approach. There are, however, other available options that contain preceding steps to performing an ABG, which are hence more suitable.

Option B: CPR should have been stopped when a valid DNAR form was found, thus you should not perpetuate further compressions.

Option C: If there is doubt about a DNAR form, for example that it cannot be found or may not be valid, then it would be appropriate to continue CPR until further information or the registrar arrives. Where there is a valid form as in this scenario, CPR should cease.

Option G: Checking the patient's pupils is a method for assessing for signs of life. However, it is initially better to assess breathing and circulation since, if they are present, then measures such as oxygen and fluids can be instigated to support them.

Option H: While stopping CPR is a good response, leaving the patient alone is not recommended. The patient may still be alive and in need of further support. The DNAR form is not a licence to stop active treatment.

Question 76

B, C, A, E, D

A career in medicine requires many compromises and is essentially a vocation which contrasts against many other traditional occupations. One such compromise is the booking of annual leave. Many constraints are placed upon arranging leave, the most important of which is conserving adequate cover to ensure patient safety. It is important to be considerate when taking leave and to consult your colleagues so that they can also enjoy their leave at convenient times.

This scenario ties together professionalism among team members and team work with maintaining a good work/life balance without threatening the care to patients. It is made more complex as the FY1 who has booked leave has not been considerate to other colleagues. This should not, however, colour your responses and the situation should be approached with consideration to both patients and the cordiality of your professional relationship with your colleagues.

Option B: The best approach would be to minimise escalation by negotiating an agreement with the FY1 at the centre of the controversy. She may not be aware of the situation that she has caused and may be amenable to rearranging her plans and leave. By speaking to her directly, you may be able to preserve the professional relationship among all of your colleagues and allow for all of you to maintain a healthy work/life balance while preventing any potential harm to patients.

Option C: Informing the consultant about the situation will allow them to intervene. The consultant is responsible for the doctors on the team and is ultimately responsible for the smooth running of the team. The consultant's intervention is likely to sour the relationship between the FY1 who has booked leave and the other colleagues. However, this is outweighed by all of the FY1s arranging convenient annual leave so that a positive work/life balance is maximised and patient safety is preserved.

Option A: Switching your on-calls with other FY1s will allow you to take leave with less inconvenience and avoids adversely affecting your relationship with the FY1 who has pre-booked leave. Conversely, this response will not help your other colleagues and still has an effect on your work/life balance. This response is subordinate to Option C due to the lower collective benefit of your actions.

Option E: This response is inappropriate given that it will sour your professional relationship with the FY1 in question with no foreseeable benefit to anyone.

Option D: Booking leave without consultation may expose patients to inadequate cover and thus risk of harm. This is the most inappropriate answer as patient safety should be your primary concern.

Question 77

E, B, C, D, A

This scenario is a common episode likely to happen during your time as an FY1. On busy firms, where consultants are not able to spend much time with patients, they may ask you to submit requests without clarifying the purpose or reason. It is important to identify in these scenarios that patient harm is a serious prospect. The 'Ionising Radiation (Medical Exposure) Regulations 2000' (IR(ME)R) state in section 2.1 that '... all medical exposures to ionising radiation must be justified prior to the exposure being made'. Should the justification not be sufficient then the harm to the patient should not be endorsed and the investigation itself may be illegal. Additionally, denying the patient the investigation, or inappropriately delaying it, may constitute harm by omission. This is of importance in this scenario, given that the question does not specify the urgency of the request. The situation is very precarious and you should not hesitate to escalate suitably.

Option E: Given that the consultant is currently busy, it would be best to approach the next senior member of the team and explain the situation. The registrar should be able to confirm the reason for the radiology request. If not, then he may be willing to approach the consultant himself.

Option B: Calling the consultant is acceptable, given that you do not know how urgent the request is. If it is very urgent, you may be exposing the patient to harm by not ensuring that it is done promptly. Second to escalating to the registrar, calling the consultant minimises the time wasted.

Option C: Asking the radiologist to intervene on your behalf is not ideal. The radiologist is likely to be busy and this may not be a good use of their time. It is selected below Option B, as it involves passing responsibility to another colleague, and inconveniencing a second person in addition to your consultant in theatre.

Option D: Delaying the request until the morning is not advisable. The urgency of the request needs to be assessed before this action is undertaken. It is safer to assume that the request is urgent rather than to delay it and risk harm to a patient, even if it means inconveniencing a radiologist and your consultant.

Option A: Deceiving the radiologist by omitting details is dishonest and contrary to GMC guidance on probity. Furthermore, lying to the radiologist may prevent them from doing their job effectively and suggesting another more appropriate investigation and thus be detrimental to the patient. Omitting clinical details may also affect the interpretation of the scan results. If it emerges that an unnecessary investigation has taken place, this is a breach of the IR(ME)R and may be illegal.

B, E, G

While hospitals endeavour to ensure that all FY1s have an equal experience and workload, this is seldom the case due to impracticality and variation between specialities. As an FY1, you are employed in a training post and learning opportunities must be grasped, however, this should not be at the cost of care to patients or to your own health or personal life. If learning opportunities are not available, this issue needs to be raised in order to safeguard your professional development and ensure that competencies are in keeping with the newer posts that you accept in future. Where you are consistently working past your hours, it is fair to chase compensation in the form of time or financial reimbursement. This is important as it has an impact on the balance between your work and personal life, and is important to maintain throughout a long career in medicine.

Option B: Addressing concerns about staffing levels is important to ensure that patients are receiving appropriate care, and to ensure that you are leaving on time to maintain a good work/life balance. Your consultant needs to be aware of the issues so that she can make provisions to resolve the situation for you and your successors.

Option E: It is a reasonable escalation to approach your educational supervisor. They may be able to help with suggestions or provide learning opportunities themselves. If the situation is particularly bad, they may intervene on your behalf and escalate further as necessary.

Option G: Going back and scrutinising the initial contract will help to ensure that you are being paid suitably. If you are working sufficiently harder and longer than your peers, then it is fair to be paid more for the additional time, in accordance with pay contracts. Alternatively, you may be offered some time off to compensate for the additional hours you have worked. This action will again help your successors as well as yourself.

Option A: This is a good response that is superseded by the options above. It is proactive to be seeking learning opportunities in order to supplement your professional development. By continuing your work as usual, you are ensuring that patient care is not further compromised by your actions. However, it fails to deal with the fact that you consistently leave late, which may have effects on patient care if the demands placed on you lead to exhaustion and burnout.

Option C: This option contrasts to Option A in the prioritisation of learning above patient care. This response is not appropriate given that your jobs for patients should be completed before looking for learning prospects.

Option D: While this response prioritises patient care in the fact that jobs are completed first, it is not ideal to compromise your personal life and time by staying back beyond hours. Continually doing so may affect your performance the next day and may eventually risk patient care.

Option F: Working harder is a short-term solution that is not sustainable. Eventually, this action will affect your overall performance and may again compromise patient care.

Option H: Complaining to the department head is a step that should follow after involving your consultant and educational supervisor and is thus superseded by other options. It is not an ideal escalation and may even be undertaken by your educational supervisor, should you approach them first.

Question 79

A, D, C, B, E

During the FY1 year you will be allocated an educational supervisor who oversees your placement both academically and professionally over the course of the year. Individual placements are managed by a separate clinical supervisor during each placement. Both supervisors will be clinicians, but the clinical supervisor will assess your clinical performance while the educational supervisor will be responsible for your development as an FY1. Both are well placed to provide assistance or advice when needed and are required to sign you off in order for you to progress in your career.

This scenario is challenging given that you are on a new placement. Most of these are for four months, and while it remains a good idea to speak to your clinical supervisor, it is noteworthy that a mid-placement review is about two months away and as such other resources should be approached. This is a suitable topic to discuss with an educational supervisor when meeting them at the start of a placement, although this is not one of the available answers for this question. In light of the options, it is necessary to deal with the matter at hand without undermining or compromising the relationship with the clinical supervisor in question.

Option A: The registrar is a good port of call. He will have experience in these matters and may know the consultant relatively well. The registrar may be able to offer guidance on how to improve or on the reasons why previous FY1s have been failed, so that you can identify areas which require improvement.

Option D: Aiming to work harder is admirable and may go some way in demonstrating that you strive to improve yourself to the consultant. Compensating for previous performance is a short-term measure, which supersedes Option C only because of the time period until your mid-placement review. This is in fact a good interim measure.

Option C: A mid-placement review will prove useful in identifying the areas that the consultant feels are weak, so that you can work on them. This will help to focus performance. Given that you have just started and currently a significant time away from a mid-placement review, interim measures such as the options above are preferred.

Option B: Avoiding your clinical supervisor attempts to avoid the issue completely. While it is not overtly dishonest, this practice is morally questionable given that patient care is likely to be interrupted. Furthermore, there is no opportunity to attempt to offer restitution for the earlier performance. This option is preferred to Option E, solely as it is more likely to preserve a good professional relationship with the clinical supervisor and does not undermine them.

Option E: Attempting to change your clinical supervisor is likely to be a difficult task as they have done nothing wrong, and it is also likely to sour your professional relationship with them.

Question 80

B, E, C, A, D

This scenario is a difficult combination of an ethical dilemma with legal consequences. While the situation itself is exaggerated considering that an FY1 is very unlikely to be faced with such specific circumstances, the teaching point remains vital.

Guidance for such dilemmas can be found predominantly in the publication 'Consent: patients and doctors making decisions together'. The salient points in this case are that the patient currently lacks capacity to make a choice given that she is unable to communicate a decision. With this in mind, you should note that the patient was not consented for an oophorectomy, and the situation has evolved whereby removing the lesion is not safe or in the patient's interests, but this is information that was not available at the time of her decision. When making decisions for patients lacking capacity, in addition to considering the patient as your first priority, 'you must also consider whether the patient's lack of capacity is temporary or permanent' and '... the views of people close to the patient on the patient's preferences, feelings, beliefs, and values'. Despite guidance that other views must be consulted and considered, the responsibility lies on the shoulders of the doctor making the decision, which should have sufficient justification. There is further guidance for times when the views of those close to the patient conflict. This guidance has not been reviewed here.

Option B: Given that removing the tumour is no longer a safe option, it would be reasonable to take a sample and send it off for histological analysis, which was within the scope of the initial procedure. As the patient's lack of capacity is temporary until the anaesthetic wears off, it would be best to allow the patient to recover before presenting her with the new information so that she can make her own informed decision.

Option E: Speaking to the patient's husband regarding his wife's probable decision will provide guidance as to what the patient might deem as acceptable. Although not the best solution, it may help to justify whatever procedure is performed given that the patient has not consented for an oophorectomy and was not aware of the risk of seeding when removing the tumour. You are not bound by the husband's information.

Option C: Performing the procedure to remove the tumour as per the previous consent risks harm that the patient was not aware of at the time of consent. This information may have coloured the patient's decision and thus performing the procedure, while partially justifiable, is not advisable. It would be pertinent to at least attempt to gauge what the patient's stance would have been in light of the changing circumstances as described in Option E.

Option A: Performing such radical surgery without consent is inappropriate. No effort has been made to uncover the patient's wishes, and she has not consented for this procedure, which is not life-saving.

Option D: Passing responsibility of the decision to be made on to the patient's husband is neglectful of your duty. While your prerogative is to act in the patient's interests, you have no guarantee that the husband does not have a conflict of interest. Although it is important to consult the husband before arriving at a decision, he should not be making the decision in your place. For this reason, this response is subordinate to Option A where a doctor is attempting to act in the patient's best interests.

Question 81

A, C, H

Breaking bad news can be a difficult task in itself and is further complicated here by the obstacles in communicating with the patient. The first major issue is whether the patient is happy to use his daughter as an interpreter. Unless he has clearly indicated consent, it would not be appropriate to employ his daughter for this purpose. The second issue is his daughter's request. Given that you cannot comply with her request, and that she may possess a conflict of interest and can regulate the flow of information which may be good or bad to her father, you should question her suitability for the role of interpreter.

GMC guidance on these two issues is quite concise. 'Good Medical Practice' states:

> You must make sure, wherever practical, that arrangements are made to meet patients' language and communication needs.

While the daughter may have been a suitable conduit previously, there are now reasons to question her ability to continue and an alternative should be considered. On the second issue, 'Treatment and care towards the end of life: good practice in decision making' instructs that:

> Apart from circumstances in which a patient refuses information, you should not withhold information necessary for making decisions (including when asked by someone close to the patient), unless you believe that giving it would cause the patient serious harm.

GMC guidance on confidentiality mentions that while you should listen to relatives should they wish to speak to you, you must endeavour to preserve the patient's confidentiality and this applies equally in this case when alluding to the patient's daughter.

Option A: Given the daughter's involvement to date, it would be best to avoid confrontation. It is, however, pertinent to explain to her that the patient will need to decide on whether he wishes to hear the information to be imparted as it may affect his further decisions on management. It is better that she knows prior to the consultation that you cannot abide by her request.

Option C: Arranging an interpreter is necessary to ensure effective communication with the patient, given that there may be concerns about the reliability of the daughter as an interpreter.

Option H: Informing your consultant about the events that have unfolded would be strongly advised. As there is potential for the daughter to complain, the consultant may wish to handle the episode differently, or even personally.

Option B: While the actions in this option are appropriate, they are superseded by the above options which deal with matters more sensitively and are less likely to inflame the situation. Where you cannot follow the daughter's request, it would be kinder to explain why than to ignore her with no explanation.

Option D: Agreeing to withhold information from the patient at the request of relatives is against GMC guidance in the absence of adequate reasoning as to why it would cause the patient serious harm.

Option E: Asking the patient whether he would like the information is ideal. This is, however, superseded by the above options because of the context of the question in which the patient does not speak English and the daughter possesses a conflict of interest which may prevent you from obtaining an honest answer to this question.

Option F: While GMC guidance does permit informing patients of the content of conversations with relatives, in this scenario doing so would not be in anyone's interests. It may create conflict between the patient and his daughter as well as among the healthcare team and the daughter. Neither would be conducive to the patient's continuing care.

Option G: Asking the daughter to leave the room is appropriate if the patient has requested it, or if you feel that her presence will undermine confidentiality. Given the daughter's closeness to the patient so far, however, it may inflame the situation to ask her to leave.

Question 82

B, D, G

In addition to a discharge summary, it is frequently necessary to provide a patient with a fit note to cover their period of illness. This is a precarious balance between providing the employer with sufficient information and not compromising the patient's confidentiality. Because of this, there is scope for abuse, particularly with the advice that the doctor may provide and the certification for the period of absence. This is obvious not only to you, but also to the patient who may identify an opportunity to extend his period of absence. It is important, therefore, that you safeguard against this and ensure that the information is both accurate and true as the custodian of this certificate. Not only is this good practice, but it is in keeping with GMC guidance in 'Good Medical Practice', which states:

> You must be honest and trustworthy when writing reports, and when completing or signing forms, reports and other documents.

At the same time, should the patient be telling the truth about his illness, you are then responsible to confirm this as his clinician such that his employment or entitlement to state welfare is not affected by genuine illness.

Option B: Completing the form for the period of illness that you are aware of is ideal. Given that you are unable to ascertain the veracity of whether the patient was truly unwell at the time of their exam, you should not include this on the fit note. If the GP is able to confirm this, it would be reasonable to ask for him to do this. It would, however, be preferable to avoid passing responsibility to the GP, when you could seek out this information yourself by contacting them directly and resolving the issue completely.

Option D: Asking the patient further questions regarding his period of sickness will help you to justify your decision and confirm facts, regardless of whether you include the two days prior to admission or choose to exclude them.

Option G: Contacting the GP minimises his workload and an unnecessary handover of responsibility to them. It also allows you to establish the facts and appropriately issue the fit note.

Option A: It would be necessary to confirm the patient's account before signing the fit note, given that you are completing a legal document upon which you are staking your honesty and reputation.

Option C: Refusing to conform to the patient's request without any justification would impact on your relationship with him. It also fails to resolve the issue and may create additional work for another healthcare professional.

Option E: There are many instances where it would be advisable to contact a senior. In this instance, contacting your registrar does not address the issue directly and is likely to result in them advising you to enact one of the above appropriate responses.

Option F: This would not be appropriate as it breaches the patient's right to confidentiality. Before making such a disclosure, it is pertinent to speak to the patient about this potential breach which is not, however, justified in this scenario.

Option H: Assessing the patient's bloods on admission does not conclusively provide a picture of their condition in the days leading up to their attendance. This does not provide good evidence that the patient was indeed ill and should not be used as justification for refusing or agreeing to add additional dates to the fit note.

Question 83

C, D, A, B, E

Answering your bleep promptly and responding to the messages that are left for you when you are not immediately available is integral to prioritising your jobs appropriately, and is good practice. You are aware that another consultant has asked for you regarding the care of one of her patients. Although you do not know whether she aims to praise, chastise or question you, it is important that you assume that the call is related to patient care. With patient care as your first priority, you must endeavour to ensure that you do not ignore the call as it may cost a patient their health or even their life.

Option C: Finding the consultant as soon as possible will enable you to find out the reason for her wish to see you. It must be assumed to be concerning patient care, perhaps to clarify the specifics of a treatment you instigated during your on-call and should be treated as so, despite the fact that it may be a routine call.

Option D: Short of finding the consultant, attempting to discover the nature of the call will help you to prioritise whether to deal with it now, or leave it until a later time.

Option A: Although not ideal, the next best thing to the above options is to contact the consultant at a later time. If the call was urgent, however, the window of opportunity to act will have been missed.

Option B: Discussing the call with your consultant is unlikely to help much at all, but is better than ignoring the call completely. There is a chance that your consultant is aware of the nature of the call, although it would be better to investigate yourself.

Option E: Ignoring the message is unprofessional. Given that you have had a hand in the patient's management, you are required to provide an adequate handover. The call may be important and you may be causing harm by not responding. This action in turn will affect the professional relationship with the consultant aiming to contact you.

Question 84

C, D, E, A, B

While it is rude to eavesdrop on a conversation among peers, if you learn of the potential for harm to a patient, it remains your duty to prevent this and safeguard the patient. In this scenario, you are faced with the prospect of clinical mishap, balanced against affecting your working relationship with peers and colleagues. Given that you have likely heard only fragments of this conversation, it would be prudent to establish the facts first, since you may have misheard information and you are not completely informed about the patient's case. Additionally, there is the teaching point about maintaining patient confidentiality and ensuring that patients and their clinical details are not identifiable in public places.

The first concern here must, as always, be the safety of the patient. Even at the detriment of your relationship with other FY1s, you must act in the patient's interests first. Of the options available, some are less likely to offend or insult your colleagues than others and thus should be selected first.

Option C: Approaching the two FY1s to inform them that there is risk of harm to the patient is the best course of action. You have dealt with matters immediately and have not overtly accused anyone of misinformation. Rather, you have suggested that it is better to consult guidance and that patient safety is at risk.

Option D: Approaching the two FY1s separately allows for a private discussion about the case and educates them that the initial course of action was incorrect. This response does not accuse one of being wrong in the presence of a peer and is less confrontational than the option below. You are less likely to cause awkwardness by telling them that they were wrong separately.

Option E: Informing both FY1s immediately that they are wrong is somewhat confrontational. This approach may cause embarrassment and could affect your working relationship with them. Since you are of the same grade, it would be more appropriate to raise concerns in a manner whereby you do not suggest that they are clearly wrong, which avoids undermining the abilities of a colleague.

Option A: Escalating the issue to the SHO should be avoided when you can directly approach the FY1s. This will be better for your professional relationship with the FY1s in question.

Option B: While patient confidentiality is important, it is subordinate to patient safety. This option is least preferred given that it does not address the issue regarding the potential for harm to a patient. In addition, the scenario is based in the staff canteen, and you are therefore likely to be in the presence of other health professionals only. It would, however, be appropriate to be wary of your surroundings when discussing confidential matters.

Question 85

C, D, E

The key to scenarios such as this is to establish whether or not the patient in question has the capacity to self-discharge or not. It is thus essential to have a reasonable awareness of the Mental Capacity Act 2005, which has been previously discussed. The salient points here are that the patient should be presumed to possess capacity. The situation is challenging as the patient is elderly and at higher risk of acute confusional states, and the patient is known to have an anxiety disorder. Despite this, there is no suggestion that the patient has impaired capacity and, as such, should be free to leave. It is important to be careful not to fall into the precaution of retaining a patient at the mention of a psychiatric illness. Anxiety disorder itself in this instance is unlikely to impair the patient's capacity to leave, and is thus not a reason to prevent a patient from discharging.

Regardless of whether the patient has capacity or not, these scenarios are always best dealt with by talking to the patient and trying to convince her to stay. In doing so, you should attempt to assess capacity briefly by asking the patient whether she understands the advantages and disadvantages of leaving. If these attempts fail and the patient does not have capacity to choose to leave, then additional action, such as using a doctor's section, may be appropriate, but this should only be used as a last resort as doing so is very likely to exacerbate the situation. At these times, obtaining senior assistance is strongly advised.

Option C: It is important to always talk to the patient in these circumstances. The reason the patient wants to leave may be a simple resolvable matter that can be easily dealt with. This would avoid the need for further escalation, whether or not the patient has capacity. The conversation itself could be directed to covertly assess capacity.

Option D: The patient should be presumed to have capacity in the absence of proof to suggest otherwise. As such, the patient is free to leave when she wishes and should be allowed to discharge. This option is second best in the absence of a response which would allow for assessment of the patient's capacity, which should be informally checked.

Option E: Given that the patient should be free to self-discharge, it would be advisable to get her to sign a form confirming that she is discharging against medical advice. This form is a legal waiver absolving the hospital of responsibility should the patient's health deteriorate. In addition, the patient should still be provided with a discharge summary where possible.

Option A: There is no indication to call a psychiatrist to come and review the patient. If a formal capacity assessment is required, then you should be able to do it yourself, provided that you have minimal training. The patient's psychiatric condition does not currently require attention.

Option B: Given that the patient is not being aggressive or violent, and that you have no grounds to hold the patient, calling security is inappropriate.

Option F: There is no reason to implement a doctor's section. There is no evidence or indication that the patient has an organic cause for acute confusion that requires either assessment or treatment.

Option G: The patient does not require sedation because there is no suggestion of risk to herself or others.

Option H: Imparting this information would be inappropriate as it is incorrect: there is no supporting evidence in the question to suggest that the patient cannot leave.

Question 86

D, C, B, E, A

The GMC states that the patient is the first concern, and that they should be listened to, with consideration paid to their views. Furthermore, every patient should be treated politely and considerately. This implies that the views of the patient with regards to their caregiver should also be respected and, as such, patients should be able to choose their doctor. Additionally, the guidance states that doctors must not unfairly discriminate against patients by allowing their personal views to adversely affect the professional relationship, or the treatment provided. These personal views include opinions on a patient's lifestyle, culture, religion or beliefs, sexual orientation, or social and economic status. Thus, decisions about a patient's management must be made on the basis of clinical judgement of their needs. Treatment cannot be withheld, especially in circumstances where a need to treat exists. Refusing to provide service in these cases will culminate in patient harm, for which you will be culpable, regardless of your personal views.

However, there is also an argument that doctors have an obligation to challenge such views and protect their colleagues from damaging remarks. Also, if an institution were to comply with an individual's request to be seen by an alternative doctor, this could result in exposure to a race discrimination claim. It is useful to seek Trust policy on racial harassment and bullying for further guidance on this issue.

In this scenario, a patient has expressed his desire to be treated by a different doctor. In the first instance, the patient's views should be explored to further understand his wishes. These may originate from a previous negative experience with a health professional from an ethnic minority. Alternatively, the patient may be reluctant to have a complex procedure performed by a junior member of staff who is relatively inexperienced. In these instances, simple reassurance may help to defuse the situation. This would also help to maintain the trust between the patient and the doctors treating him. Where a patient continues to refuse to have treatment from a particular doctor, for whatever reason, alternative measures should be arranged to prevent them from coming to harm. Trust policy may vary on this issue, from refusing all but emergency treatment, to complete refusal of treatment.

Option D: Exploring the patient's views will help to determine the reasons why the patient is reluctant to have the procedure performed by your colleague. This may uncover reasons which could be addressed through reassurance.

Option C: If the patient continues to refuse to be seen by your colleague, he cannot be treated against his wishes. It would be pertinent to handle the situation with your colleague sensitively and provide him with adequate support and explain the situation. Efforts should also be made to reassure the patient about your colleague's abilities, with the aim of maintaining the patient's faith in the healthcare team.

Option B: Trust policy may vary regarding whether or not further treatment is provided. With reference to the GMC guidance stated above, arranging for the procedure to be performed by another colleague should proceed if this is deemed to be in the patient's best interests.

Option E: The GMC states that patient's views must be respected. While an argument could be made that the reasons for choosing to be treated by another doctor are flawed, it would be unusual to dissuade him unless his choice was detrimental to his health. There are, however, instances where such preferences are acceptable. Patients may have appropriate and legitimate reasons for choosing a doctor on the basis of their gender or religion; a female patient may prefer to be seen by a clinician of the same sex for an intimate examination. The clinician must endeavour to meet the patient's wishes in such instances.

Option A: This is the least appropriate option. While Trust policy may vary regarding how much treatment the patient is afforded, there may be a need to treat him in an emergency situation if his condition deteriorates. This response also goes against GMC guidance about patients not being judged by the views they hold.

Question 87

A, B, F

The GMC publication 'Confidentiality' aptly summarises the stance that 'Your duty of confidentiality continues after a patient has died'. The same paragraph highlights that patients' wishes should be respected after death, in the case that they have asked for specific information to remain confidential. When making disclosures, you should consider the nature of the content that is to be disclosed, the effect the information will have on the family and whether the information is already in the public domain or not. There is scope to inform relatives of the cause of death, or the events in the run-up to the patient's death 'when a partner, close relative or friend asks for information about the circumstances of an adult's death, and you have no reason to believe that the patient would have objected to such a disclosure'. When in doubt, it is better not to make any disclosures and to consult a senior with greater experience.

Option A: Given that you are unaware of the relative's request or the information that they seek, it is advisable to inform them that there is a possibility that you cannot provide the information in the interests of the deceased party.

Option B: Asking a senior colleague in this instance is a reasonable escalation. Scenarios around confidentiality can be very complicated and unsolicited information may have legal consequences. You may benefit from senior experience and will be able to discuss any areas that you must not disclose to the relatives on the patient's request.

Option F: Finding out what the family wish to know will help you to judge whether or not you are able to make the disclosure. It is important to assess the nature and quantity of the information that the family seek before disclosing anything.

Option C: Telling the family that you cannot impart the information is not a good answer as you cannot ascertain the veracity of the statement. As you do not know the information that the family are requesting, you cannot judge whether or not to tell them anything.

Option D: Asking the ward sister to speak to the relatives is effectively shirking your responsibilities. Part of your duty is to speak to families, and you should not be passing on this responsibility without good reason.

Option E: While the staff at the bereavement office are better versed in talking to families after death, it is not ideal to refer to them so early after the death. They may not be as familiar with the patient or the family as you and may not be in as good a position to deal with the request, given that you remain unaware of why the relatives wish to speak to you.

Option G: Asking for a senior colleague to talk to the family is reasonable given the potential complications of an improper disclosure of information. It is superseded by Option B though, because obtaining advice and speaking to the family yourself would suffice rather than shifting responsibility onto someone else. If you continue to remain uncomfortable about the situation, it may be necessary to request the involvement of a senior colleague.

Option H: Similarly to Option C, as you are unaware of the information that the relatives seek, you cannot disclose the details. The suitability of this option depends on the nature of the information requested.

Question 88

A, C, D

Testing scenarios in which an element of trust is placed in a patient, who has made the same promises in the past, can be at times very frustrating. It is imperative when managing such patients that you remain non-judgemental and objective. Where your concerns are objectively serious, as in this situation, you need to ensure that you act in the patient's best interests. In this case, prescribing metronidazole may actually cause harm and may not help with the tooth abscess. It is better thus to search for an alternative where possible. It is not that you disbelieve the patient but that you are preparing for things not going according to plan. The patient needs to be made fully aware of the consequences of breaching the instructions given, so that his choice to drink on the medication is fully informed. This is especially important if an alternative cannot be found and the patient ultimately has to be discharged on the original antibiotic. It is not acceptable to discharge the patient without treatment because you do not trust him, as this may in fact cause harm by omission.

Option A: Ensuring that the advice given to the patient is on the discharge summary means that the GP will be aware of what has happened as an inpatient. It is also a point of reference for the patient and legal documentation of your actions, which can be used in your defence if the patient does not heed the instructions he has agreed to follow.

Option C: Informing the patient not to take the antibiotic if he is drinking is important safety-net advice. The side-effects can be severe and cause serious distress. In this way, the harm caused can be limited and this may in fact be an opportunity for the patient to seek further medical advice. With this option, you are attempting to treat the patient and are limiting the potential harm.

Option D: Consulting the microbiology consultant will help to optimise the treatment so as to again limit the risk of harm from an interaction. This may minimise the effect of taking the drug for the patient and would be precautionary in the case that he continues drinking.

Option B: Informing the patient that he is responsible for his actions, after informing him of the potential effects, is acceptable. It does not, however, help to minimise the risk of an interaction or does not offer advice. Thus it is less suitable than the responses above.

Option E: Discharging the patient without antibiotics will not treat his underlying condition. This response will likely cost him the loss of his tooth, as well as the risk of sepsis. Despite the patient's history, he has given assurances that should be respected. While he will be responsible for the harm of not listening to your advice, you will be liable for the harm resulting from the untreated abscess.

Option F: Since the patient has stated that he will not drink alcohol while on metronidazole, there is no reason to believe that prescribing it is guaranteed to cause harm. The patient is aware of the consequences and, although it would be wiser to prescribe an alternate antibiotic, it would be appropriate to discharge him with metronidazole.

Option G: Asking the patient's wife to monitor her husband would be unfairly passing on responsibility. Furthermore, it may breach the patient's confidentiality if he is unaware of the disclosure.

Option H: Giving the patient an additional medication such as acamprosate is not advisable given that this is not an indication to prescribe, and is unlikely to work.

Question 89

E, D, B, C, A

It is not unusual for patients to make requests that compromise the professionalism of your practice, and place you in the middle of a medico-legal or ethical dilemma. In this question, you are being asked to weigh a patient's confidentiality against probity, which is expected of doctors, and in this case demanded by your employer.

The issue of confidentiality is covered extensively elsewhere in this book, however, the salient details are that you cannot break confidentiality unless the patient gives permission. It is made more complex as sufficient justification to break confidentiality without consent is not present here. Additionally, it must be borne in mind that 'Good Medical Practice' states, on the matter of probity:

> You must do your best to make sure that any documents you write or sign are not false or misleading. This means that you must take reasonable steps to verify the information in the documents, and that you must not deliberately leave out relevant information.

However, in support of omitting details, it also states elsewhere that:

> ... you should tell the general practitioner the results of the investigations, the treatment provided or any other information necessary for the continuing care of the patient, unless the patient objects.

Thus the patient's wishes need to be honoured.

Given the intricacy of this matter, as the patient's demands place you in a difficult ethical position affecting your probity and compromising your contracted duty to ensure the hospital must be paid, it is important to escalate the matter early. If you cannot persuade the patient to change his stance, then your seniors should be informed before you proceed with further actions that may compromise either your employment, or alternatively, your duties as a doctor.

Option E: Talking to the patient about his request may uncover the reason and may allow you to address the issue, preventing the need for further action. It will give you an insight into the patient's thinking and will enable both you and your seniors to make a better informed decision.

Option D: Informing a senior early is important in complex scenarios where you cannot resolve the situation. Having sanction from a senior will help to protect your position in whatever further action is taken, given that all the options threaten your position. There may be measures in place to ensure the hospital receives reimbursement without the knowledge of the GP.

Option B: Omitting the details, while not ideal, protects the patient's confidentiality and is in keeping with GMC guidance. It is subordinate to the above responses as it prevents the GP providing optimum care, which may be achieved with Option E, and also compromises your duty to the hospital.

Option C: Ignoring the patient's request means breaking confidentiality. This is improper and is bad practice. It will affect your professional relationship with the patient and cannot be justified in this scenario.

Option A: Breaking the patient's confidentiality is not appropriate, but is made worse by not informing him prior to doing so and in effect deceiving him. This action will threaten the trust the patient has in both you and the profession. It is worse than Option C, involving underhand tactics in addition to neglecting your duty to the patient.

Question 90

E, B, A, C, D

Doctors are in a privileged position with their patients and share a unique relationship with them. The GMC recognises that such affiliations are based on openness, trust and good communication, and enables doctors to work in partnership with their patients to address their individual needs. Often patients are in a vulnerable position and this responsibility must be managed carefully to ensure that it is not exploited. The GMC states:

> You must not use your professional position to establish or pursue a sexual or improper emotional relationship with a patient or someone close to them.

It is important to establish the facts and not jump to conclusions about what has been observed. The patient in this scenario may be distressed after having received bad news or having difficulty coping, with the doctor empathetically supporting them. Speaking to a trusted senior colleague may provide insight into what you have seen, and they may be in a better position to determine whether it is appropriate and reassure you that this is your consultant's regular bedside manner when dealing with a distressed patient.

This scenario does not provide sufficient evidence to conclude that there is anything untoward, or that an obvious breach of guidelines has occurred. In such instances, it is important to act as it may undermine public confidence or put the medical profession in disrepute. Supplementary guidance from the GMC acknowledges that:

> In most successful doctor–patient relationships a professional boundary exists between doctor and patient. If this boundary is breached, this can undermine the patient's trust in their doctor, as well as the public's trust in the medical profession.

Option E: It is important not to assume that the consultant has behaved inappropriately based on what you have seen. Tactful questioning may help to uncover what has happened; the patient may have required extra support through a difficult time, and the consultant may have a long-standing, established professional relationship with them. Such action should be performed delicately to avoid confrontation, which will adversely affect your working relationship with the consultant.

Option B: Speaking to a trusted colleague, such as your registrar, may provide a different perspective on what you have seen. He may have more experience on your consultant's regular manner with patients and would be able to judge what is appropriate. He may also be able to provide you with support if further action is required.

Option A: Asking the patient to leave immediately will harm your relationship with the consultant and may impact upon the trust the patient has in the healthcare team. It may be insulting to the patient and your senior colleague, particularly if your consultant is providing the patient with support and reassurance. It may, however, be necessary in order to deal with the issue if there is reason to believe that this is an improper relationship.

Option C: This would be an inappropriate escalation without first establishing the facts and allowing the consultant to explain his actions. This will also impact on the relationship you have with the consultant.

Option D: Doing nothing is the least appropriate response. If there is a potential breach of guidelines, you cannot ignore the issue.

Question 91

B, E, F

Issues surrounding domestic violence can be challenging to deal with. The nature of the doctor–patient relationship allows for sensitive information to be shared in confidence. There are instances, however, where this agreement must be broken. Victims of abuse are within their rights to request that their personal information is not disclosed to other groups. Encouraging victims to take action against such abuse can be difficult as there are many practical and emotional barriers to leaving a violent partner. These range from housing and money, to protecting children that are involved, and an attachment or fear of their partner. The fact that children are also subject to abuse, however, changes how the situation should be dealt with. There is a need to break confidentiality where there are child protection issues. In this scenario, the partner is abusive with both his wife and child. If a child is being put at risk, you must act.

Option B: It would be appropriate for social services to be involved in this scenario, and they will be able to provide advice and take the relevant action to ensure that the child is safeguarded. This should ideally be performed once the situation has been explained to the patient and consent to disclosure has been sought. However, there is a need to contact social services even without consent, in order to protect the child that is involved. This action may not necessarily involve the child being taken away from the couple, but will ensure that they are safe.

Option E: Speaking to a senior colleague will keep them informed of the situation and allow them to advise you on the appropriate action. Their experience will help to ensure that the scenario is dealt with carefully and sensitively.

Option F: This response will inform the patient of the options that are available and may help her to leave her abusive partner. While this does not deal with the needs of the child or the child protection issue directly, which are your top priority, it would be more appropriate than contacting the police.

Option A: This response passes responsibility to another colleague, whereas it would be more appropriate for you to act. There are no assurances that the case will be followed up and leaves both the patient and child exposed to further harm.

Option C: Informing the abusive partner potentially puts both the patient and child at risk of reprisals. There is no guarantee that the partner will attend and it may worsen the situation.

Option D: The abusive partner may not attend the appointment that you make. This request may also raise suspicions, particularly as his wife has only recently been treated by you at the hospital. This could potentially put the patient and child at risk.

Option G: Although the patient does not wish for any action to be taken, you must act since the child is being put at risk.

Option H: The patient does not wish for any further action to be taken, and informing the police is unlikely to benefit the situation, since as far as you can assess there is no immediate danger. The police will contact social services, and it would be more appropriate for you to do this yourself. While it may be necessary to inform the police at some stage, there are more immediate actions that should be undertaken.

Question 92

D, A, C, E, B

All members of the healthcare team have a duty to behave professionally and maintain trust in the profession. However, outside of work there should be a remit to enjoy oneself and have a healthy personal life. There are some caveats to this; if the actions of a colleague pose a potential risk to patients, this cannot be ignored and appropriate action should be taken. This would include the use of illicit drugs or viewing child pornography, as these may result in patient harm. In this scenario, patient safety is not at risk and therefore no action is needed. Further, any action that is undertaken is likely to adversely affect the relationship you have with your colleagues.

Option D: Patient safety is not at risk, and so no action is needed. The remaining responses are all inappropriate and are ranked in the order of increasing escalation.

Option A: There is no need to speak to the nurse privately as she has not done anything wrong. When there are issues which need to be discussed, dealing with problems locally before escalating appropriately is advised.

Option C: Informing the entire group of nurses that their actions are wrong will harm the working relationship you have with them. This is especially so, given that they have not done anything wrong.

Option E: The ward sister is the next professional up in the hierarchy. Informing a senior colleague may be necessary in instances of wrong-doing. The ward sister is involved in the training of nursing staff and would be more appropriate to inform than the consultant.

Option B: Doctors frequently have a role as heads of the healthcare team, where they are required to lead and manage all professionals to optimise patient care. Informing the consultant would therefore constitute the highest level of escalation given the options available.

Question 93

A, C, B, D, E

It is inadvisable to influence the management of a patient that is not under the care of your team, unless in an emergency situation. Nurses may approach you, however, with requests for patients that are not your own, when the regular team is off the ward. Without knowing the specific details of the patient's management it is not appropriate to intervene. When you are on-call, you have a duty to cover all patients while the regular teams are not available. However, this is not the case during a regular working day.

Despite the team's management, it may be acceptable to restart a patient on analgesia that has been recently stopped if the weaning process has been titrated prematurely. With this in mind, it is unclear whether harm has come to the patient or not.

Option A: With patients remaining your first concern, it would be appropriate to ensure that no harm has come to them and to treat and reverse any issues that may have arisen due to your actions.

Option C: Keeping the regular team informed is important so that they can adapt the patient's management plan accordingly. They will be best placed to determine the most appropriate subsequent steps.

Option B: While confronting the nurse is not ideal, it supersedes the responses below. It is better to calmly discuss the nurse's actions with her to understand the rationale. Confronting the nurse may affect your working relationship with her but allows for reflection on this episode and a modified approach to future instances where a patient requires a doctor's attention.

Option D: This would not be appropriate, as there is no confirmation of patient harm. Apologising to the patient inappropriately may in fact shake their confidence in the healthcare team and affect their relationship with the team normally looking after them. If patient harm was confirmed, it would then be appropriate to provide a prompt and honest explanation as per GMC guidance. Harming the relationship between the patient and the healthcare team is more serious than affecting that between you and the nurse, and as such this response ranks below Option B.

Option E: This is not advisable as the analgesic may require a weaning process, and immediately stopping the drug may cause the patient harm. Careful consideration should be made before any rash action. Additionally, withholding the analgesic may cause the pain to return and remain uncontrolled. You should refrain from further involvement in the patient's management and allow the regular team to make better informed decisions concerning the patient's care. While this option is not in itself a bad response, it is superseded by the responses above which would be more appropriate in this scenario.

Question 94

C, D, G

You may frequently find that patients ask you a question to which you are unaware of the answer. The patient may assume that your knowledge encompasses a sufficient breadth of medicine and surgery in order to provide reliable and accurate responses. Admitting ignorance in this scenario can make for a difficult encounter. This scenario requires a balance between ensuring probity and the amount of trust that a patient places in your ability. It is imperative that you do not provide false or misleading information which may affect the informed consent that the patient is later to provide. This includes speculating or extrapolating the details of a procedure and presenting it as fact.

In these instances, it is most appropriate to either defer to a more experienced colleague or to acquire this information yourself and present it to the patient. It is important to be mindful of how this information is presented to ensure that it does not compromise their belief in the procedure or the surgeons involved.

Option C: This option shows the patient that you are attempting to find out the information that she requires and deals with her concerns. It therefore directly deals with the issues that the patient has raised. However, it indirectly informs her that you do not have an understanding of the procedure in question. This may affect the belief that the patient places in your ability, though it is clear that you will not be performing the operation.

Option D: Asking a senior colleague will deal with the patient's concerns and ensure that she does not have a nasty surprise on the morning of the procedure when she is consented for it. While the escalation can be avoided, it will reaffirm the patient's confidence in the hierarchy of care, at the calculated cost of the patient's impression of your ability.

Option G: Reviewing the clinic letters in the patient's notes will enable you to appreciate her presenting complaint and the circumstances leading up to her admission for elective surgery. Correspondence by more senior members of your team will discuss the various management options, and the details of and justification for surgery. This can be interpreted for the patient in order to ensure that she is aware of what the surgery will aim to achieve. This also enables you to tailor the information you provide so that it is relevant for the patient, as opposed to Option E, where the information is likely to be more generic.

Option A: Extrapolating what you believe the procedure to involve provides the patient with an answer that is not based upon fact. There is no guarantee that your answer is accurate and it may have the consequence of the patient refusing the operation on the day of the procedure when she learns that it is not what she was expecting.

Option B: Responding to the patient's concerns on the day of surgery is not appropriate, as she may then refuse to have the operation on the basis that she did not anticipate the type of surgery that has been scheduled. There is no guarantee that the issues will be addressed on a busy morning ahead of an operating list. It also defers responsibility to another colleague who may not have time to address these concerns in the process of consenting all the patients on the day's operating list.

Option E: Directing the patient to a reliable website is a reasonable answer superseded by Option C. It is better for you to learn about the procedure yourself and ensure the patient's understanding, rather than leaving her to her own devices where she may encounter less relevant information, have further questions or misinterpret the information published.

Option F: Telling the patient that you do not know what the procedure involves does not deal with the patient's concerns. It may also compromise her faith in the care that you provide.

Option H: There is no reason to believe that the patient is likely to withhold consent. Furthermore, this appointment is only to assess the patient's fitness for surgery, something that will still have to be done at another time if the operation is to proceed, potentially delaying surgery. You are not dealing with the patient's query and will have wasted both her time and yours.

Question 95

C, A, E, D, B

Encouraging or assisting suicide is a criminal offence in the UK. The GMC states that doctors must 'show respect for human life' and 'follow the law that affects their practice and ensure that their conduct at all times justifies their patients' trust in them and public trust in the profession'. There is a potential conflict of interest in these instances. While doctors must make care of patients their first priority, they should respect the competent patient's right to refuse treatment, even if this will lead to their death. However, doctors must continue to provide whatever care is accepted and ensure that their actions or advice do not encourage or assist suicide. It is important to understand the needs of patients and respect their privacy and dignity. Guidance issued by the GMC states:

> *Where patients raise the issue of assisted suicide, or ask for information that might encourage or assist them in ending their lives, doctors should explain that they cannot do so because providing this information would mean breaking the criminal law.*

Option C: You must assess the patient for depression and complete a suicide risk assessment on her. It would be appropriate to assess her fully before a judgement is made about her mood and treatment started.

Option A: Involving a psychiatrist may help to establish whether the patient is depressed and determine the risk to herself (and others). This is important should the psychiatrist wish to follow up the patient in the community and ensure that she is safe to be discharged if appropriate. This response is subordinate to the option above as you should not assume that a patient is depressed before an assessment is made.

Option E: It is a criminal offence to provide any kind of assistance to a patient who wishes to die. This includes giving help and advice on assisted suicide clinics abroad. This response is preferred to those below, which include measures to help the patient die, as opposed to simply providing information.

Option D: It is illegal to assist a patient to die. If a patient is assessed as having capacity and refuses treatment, then you must respect their wishes. It is not clear in this question whether the patient has capacity or not and there is no mention of a refusal to accept treatment. If a patient does have capacity, and makes an undesirable choice regarding their treatment, you must ensure that they are aware of the potential consequences of their decision. In this response, you are specifically withholding treatment with no specific refusal of treatment from the patient, with the view of passively assisting suicide.

Option B: This is the least appropriate response as active measures are taken to assist with suicide. This is illegal and is likely to result in criminal proceedings.

Question 96

B, D, H

It is a significant challenge when you are approached with a problem which lies out of the realms of medical science, within the parameters of a social problem, about which you know little. The available responses in this question include many sensible options, however, it is better to clarify the situation with the best information available.

It would be incorrect to assume that the knowledge you possess about the patient's religion is accurate and presumption may offend the patient. In this scenario, it is clear that the patient is not medically fit to fast. It is thus in his medical interests to persuade him not to fast. This may be as simple as presenting the patient with the risks and potential effects of the religious observance, but may require ingenuity in obtaining the facts about the religion and the stance on obeying medical advice. Given that different sects and belief systems exist in all religions, and that you cannot know them all, it is better that you enable the patient to find the information himself.

Should the patient remain adamant that he wants to fast, it then becomes a question of minimising the risk of harm, where you cannot prevent it. In this case, you should attempt to modify his regime as best as possible and weigh the risks of potential hypoglycaemic episodes against the detriment of persistently high blood glucose. Even when adapting medical therapy, you should endeavour to find out from the patient what options are permissible and which are not, during the observance of the fast.

Option B: It is first pertinent to inform the patient about what you know to be true. In this case, he needs to know that it would be harmful to his health to fast with poorly controlled diabetes. This ensures the patient is fully informed and may help to persuade the patient not to fast.

Option D: Asking the patient about what the religion says in the face of medical advice is a good response. Regardless of your level of knowledge on the issue, you should attempt to elicit the patient's individual understanding of his beliefs. This may provide suitable reasoning, which is supported by religious teachings, on the need to prioritise his health over observing his beliefs which may compromise his well-being. Alternatively, it may alert you early on in the consultation that your medical advice will not dissuade the patient, and appropriate supportive strategies are required to allow the patient to fast while minimising the risk to himself. It is important to note that this consultation should not challenge his beliefs, and that you must work with the patient to reach a mutually agreeable management plan.

Option H: An alternative to Option D, telling the patient to gather information on the prospect of not fasting may convince the patient to follow medical advice or prevent you from an act of futility, in which you try to convince the patient to avoid keeping this religious observance.

Option A: Offering medical advice to minimise risk at this stage is premature, when you should aim to avoid the risk of harm altogether. The medical advice itself in this option is not sound either, as without insulin, the patient risks a life-threatening episode of diabetic ketoacidosis.

Option C: Phoning the local religious leader may not be the patient's religious leader and may offer advice that does not apply. It is thus better to let the patient source his own information. Furthermore, if the patient is known to the religious leader, the limited information you provide may still lead to him being identified, compromising confidentiality.

Option E: Asking a more experienced GP to help is a good option. It is, however, superseded by the above options because they are actions that the GP will likely undertake, which you can do yourself before approaching the GP.

Option F: Modifying the regime is a good option that should be the last step if you fail to convince the patient to avoid fasting. It is thus subordinate to the correct responses above.

Option G: It is reasonable to offer the patient this advice but it is better to first try to prevent harm altogether and convince the patient to avoid fasting. It is important to know more about the observance and the religion. It could well be the case that the patient's beliefs do not permit him to check his blood glucose levels when fasting.

Question 97

C, B, D, E, A

This scenario assesses your ability to prioritise your work/life balance against your duty to patients. In accordance with GMC guidance, patients must remain your top concern. Remaining in hospital to ensure that the appropriate emergency treatment is provided is therefore essential. Should you need to leave, you must ensure that an adequate handover has taken place and not leave this in the trust of another health professional.

Option C: With patients as your top priority, it is important to ensure that the necessary treatment is initiated promptly. Despite the fact that your shift has ended, you must provide adequate immediate management before handing over which is likely to delay treatment.

Option B: Contacting the on-call team ensures that they are aware of the patient and enables them to take over the patient's management.

Option D: Requesting that the nurse contacts the on-call team does not guarantee that this task will be completed with due urgency. A nurse to doctor handover is also not as appropriate as a handover from yourself, which would ensure the relevant details are imparted and the urgency of the situation is communicated.

Option E: This would not be appropriate as it fails to deal with the urgency of the situation. It is, however, more appropriate than the response below, as it aims to address the problem. It is inferior to Option D, where there remains a possibility for prompt treatment to be initiated by the on-call team if the nurse makes contact with them. A review in the morning allows for the patient to be assessed and treatment initiated, albeit delayed.

Option A: Berating the nurse does not deal with the patient, who must remain your priority. It also adversely affects your working relationship with the nurse. It would be more appropriate to have a private discussion with her to address your grievances, although this should take place once you have dealt with the patient.

Question 98

A, B, D, E, C

Approaching your colleagues about sensitive issues must be done tactfully if it is to avoid causing offence or harm your working relationship with him. In exploring this issue, any precipitating factors may be uncovered which you may be able to help with, or provide support for. Your colleague may be experiencing personal problems which may account for the deterioration in self-care. If it is not an issue that affects patient care, there is no priority for you to act. It is also important to protect the working relationship of other members of the healthcare team that may be involved. It is therefore essential that you do not disclose the identities of anyone who has raised concerns regarding the issue, since they have approached you in confidence.

Option A: Your colleague's recent change in self-care may stem from an issue in his personal life. It is best dealt with by discussing this with him and uncovering if there is an issue with which you can offer assistance. If there is a problem in his personal life, there may be a need for it to be addressed to avoid an impact upon patient care. It may be the case that there is a reasonable explanation for the change that your colleague is unaware of, such as cycling into work, which may be resolved by simply highlighting this to him.

Option B: Involving your registrar would enable an experienced member of the team to intervene and address the issue. However, this would be an inappropriate escalation with an issue that you could potentially address yourself. Involving your registrar spares your working relationship with your colleague, in contrast to the responses below.

Option D: As patient care is not compromised by the issue, there is no urgency for you to act. Doing nothing is more appropriate than the responses below, as there is scope for working relationships to be negatively impacted by these actions.

Option E: While you may have good intentions, gifting your colleague self-care products may be misinterpreted by him. This is likely to adversely affect your working relationship with him. It would be more appropriate to address the issue directly by having a private discussion with your colleague, rather than to offer subtle hints which may not work or may cause offence.

Option C: Informing your colleague about who has raised concerns about his body odour is inappropriate. This action may have ramifications on your relationship with the ward sister, who is less likely to approach you in confidence, as well as her relationship with your colleague, who may take offence at her not approaching him directly or raising the issue in the first place.

B, E, H

It is very difficult to challenge a senior in a position of authority given that he is responsible for your practice and for your development as a doctor. While you do work for your consultant, you are officially employed by the hospital to look after NHS patients, and are thus not employed to look after your consultant's private patients unless instructed by your employer. This scenario presents a risk to all the patients through compromised care as your duties accumulate. It is important to remember that patient safety is the first concern and, although you will have to work for both sets of patients in the immediate setting, you must recognise that this is not a long-term solution.

Resolving this situation is impossible without either confronting the consultant or escalating the matter to someone else. Bypassing the consultant and escalating to another may unnecessarily inflame the situation and damage your working relationship. The first port of call should thus be speaking to him directly but as he is partly responsible for your progression, approaching him must be done with tact. Should this fail, seeking advice or further escalating the matter needs to be considered.

Option B: Patient care and safety should always come first. You cannot discriminate against groups of patients for any reason, and as such should attend to them and their jobs in order of necessity, dealing with the more urgent jobs first. This is not an ideal long-term solution, but is required in the interim.

Option E: This is a good solution in the interim, given the importance of patient care. When normally performing a test, you are responsible for either verifying the results or handing over that they require checking. By delegating part of the task to the consultant for his own patients, you are freeing yourself to provide better care for all of the patients.

Option H: Confronting your consultant is essential to stop this situation perpetuating. It is preferred to involving others as it deals with the issue more directly and will have less of an impact on your working relationship.

Option A: Prioritising your own patients over the private patients is ill advised and may lead to harm if you unwittingly neglect an urgent duty. The potential for patient harm makes this option inappropriate, even though you are not employed to look after the private patients.

Option C: Speaking to your registrar may help as they will be able to advise you on how you should proceed. Despite being a good response, patient care must come first and, furthermore, it is preferred to speak to the consultant directly before involving another party.

Option D: Similarly to Option C, this is an appropriate response which should, however, be delayed in the interests of patient care and the working relationship with the consultant.

Option F: Refusing to provide care for the private patients may place them at risk of harm. Thus this action is not recommended.

Option G: This option opens the prospect of patient harm by neglecting a patient in distress by irresponsibly prioritising jobs.

Question 100

D, B, A, E, C

Given the vast array of medication and alternative drugs that are available for use, it is unlikely that you will have a full appreciation of every medicine. The production process of drugs is not common knowledge and very few doctors are likely to know intricate details such as the porcine origin of enoxaparin.

It is important to respect the religious beliefs held by patients, and to gain consent for treatment. While it is reasonable to assume implied consent every time the patient rolls up her top for her injection to the abdomen, she needs to be fully informed of her decision. Given that you are now aware of information that may change her decision, it would be pertinent to put the information to the patient so that she can re-evaluate. At the same time, you should not assume familiarity with the patient's religion. While some Muslims may believe items which are forbidden become permissible as medical treatment, others do not. Thus, it would be best to discuss these beliefs with the patient herself. Furthermore, just because the patient's son objects to the treatment, it does not mean that the patient shares his beliefs.

Although it is not presented here as an option, it would be advisable to notify a senior member of the team about the events which have unfolded. Before proceeding further, you should verify that the information is in fact true. It is ultimately the patient's decision as to whether she would like enoxaparin or not, and you should be aware that facilities such as a Muslim chaplain may exist at the hospital, and that they may be able to offer some advice.

Option D: It is the patient's decision as to whether or not they receive the enoxaparin. It is ideal to tell the patient of the new information that you have gathered as you have a reason to believe that it may affect her decision. Additionally, you may wish to outline the risks of refusing enoxaparin. Ultimately, you must follow your patient's instruction about the enoxaparin.

Option B: The prescription of enoxaparin confers benefit that is judged to be greater than the risks of not receiving it. If the patient has not objected to its use, it should be continued as stopping it puts her at risk of deep vein thrombosis (DVT). Given that you do not know whether or not the patient is Muslim or the beliefs that she holds, the enoxaparin should be continued. It would, however, be advisable to speak to her son about her beliefs concerning enoxaparin, given its origin, if it is not possible to talk to her directly.

Option A: Giving a less effective alternative is not ideal unless you have established that the patient objects to the use of enoxaparin. This option is superior to those below, given that the patient's son's personal beliefs should not affect her treatment, and that it is better than no treatment at all.

Option E: Exploring the son's beliefs about treatment is not of much use given that there is no guarantee that the patient herself holds the same values. As such, it would be irresponsible to base management decisions on the outcome of this discussion. It would be better to speak to the son regarding what his mother believes, and any previous decisions or preferences she has expressed.

Option C: Actively withdrawing the enoxaparin, which is of medical benefit, without the patient's express instruction is most likely to cause harm. This option is more acceptable if either the patient or her son had expressed that enoxaparin is not compatible with the patient's values.

Question 101

A, C, B, D, E

There will be instances where the procedures you attempt on patients are unsuccessful, and there is a need to seek further assistance. Communicating with patients about the reasons why it is necessary will ensure that they are kept informed of its necessity. There must be a balance between the continued harm of repeated attempts, against the benefits of the treatment they are to receive. Escalation should follow a hierarchical chain and where not possible, alternative approaches should be weighed against the need for the procedure.

Option A: Although protocol varies between Trusts, repeated failed attempts should prompt escalation to your immediate senior. Calling a more experienced colleague also has the benefit of a second opinion on further management of the patient; the SHO may provide insight into the urgency of the cannula, whether it can wait for the regular team and the possibility of switching to oral antibiotics.

Option C: As the cannula is being used to provide the patient with antibiotics and fluids, it can be deemed to be important and of benefit to the patient in the absence of further information. Calling the anaesthetist in moments of difficult but necessary cannulation is acceptable in cases where the chain of escalation has been exhausted.

Option B: When it has not been possible to site the cannula, or the above options are not available, alternatives to the cannula must be sought. Given that the patient requires antibiotics, it is pertinent to provide something in the form of oral antibiotics even if it is subordinate to the intravenous form. The day team can then reattempt or reassess the need for a cannula later.

Option D: Waiting on the patient's day team to take care of the situation is neglecting your duty of care to the patient. It is important to at least attempt to insert a cannula if it is required or to provide an interim alternative where not possible. Not receiving any care may be harmful to the patient. This response supersedes Option E, where you do not have consent to perform the procedure and are going against the patient's wishes.

Option E: Attempting to site a cannula in the patient's leg even though he has refused would constitute assault. When other options have been exhausted and the cannula is required, it would be pertinent to ensure that the patient is fully informed regarding their refusal and the effects of not receiving treatment.

Question 102

A, E, H

GMC guidance applies both to doctors and medical students alike. The student in this scenario has contravened GMC guidance on probity, given that he has written an essay that is plagiarised and has attempted to pass it off as his own. However, it is important to note that his conduct is not a risk to patient safety, and neither has he done anything to compromise patient care.

In an instance where you are aware that a doctor has published material claiming credit for another's work, you should escalate according to local policy. If the subject is not addressed by local policy, it may be necessary to escalate the matter to the deanery or, if appropriate, further still to the GMC. However, when escalating such an issue, an element of reasonable personal judgement should be used since there is no concrete official guidance on this topic. Specifically, you must weigh the need to escalate this matter and its seriousness against the potential harm to the profession from making an accusation, and the effect it will have on patients' trust in doctors. Furthermore, such accusations should not be made without significant reason, given that colleagues should be afforded respect.

In this situation, where a student has presented an essay before submission, it can be argued that he has not plagiarised any material yet. Furthermore, given that you are a member of the team responsible for his education, your actions constitute a level of escalation in themselves. It may be the case that you have seen a draft copy and that the student intends to make further modifications to the text including proper referencing. He also may not be aware of the GMC guidance on probity. In this case, you must ensure that he is aware of the rules that he is breaking, to improve his future practice and conduct. It is also important to afford him reasonable guidance and the benefit of the doubt given that he has not officially submitted anything. With this in mind, you should try not to act prematurely with actions that may stain his medical student career and by extension his further practice.

Option A: Asking the student to rewrite the essay before submission will give him an opportunity to correct his errors. As a member of the team responsible for his education, this action may be considered as part of the reprimand for plagiarism. While having to review the student's work again will cost you some of your time, it will ensure that you have taught the student and he has understood how his actions constituted plagiarism and how this is to be avoided.

Option E: This should be the first action. Speaking to the student will uncover what his intentions are. It may be that he has copied this source with the intention of later referencing it, or intends to check with you that he has found a good source. Understanding why the material has been copied will help to decide on further action.

Option H: The student may not be aware that his essay in its current state undermines GMC guidance on probity. Explaining this to him is important as it is the issue at hand and may prevent him from doing this in future as a doctor and improve his future conduct.

Option B: Not acting on your discovery is not appropriate. Given that the student is your tutee, you should at least endeavour to find out whether he is aware of what he has done and tell him why it is wrong. Educating him is part of your duty in this role, especially as you have agreed to review the document already. By allowing him to submit such a document, knowing its faults, without at least informing him of GMC guidance on the matter, would be neglecting the trust he places in you and would be unbecoming of a doctor.

Option C: Informing the consultant at this point would be premature. The student has yet to submit the document and is asking you to review it in trust. By informing the consultant at this early stage, you may affect the opinion that the consultant has of the student and consequently affect the manner in which his work is marked.

Option D: Speaking to the consultant in private is appropriate, despite being superseded by the options above. Asking the consultant's advice is a good response, given that there is no formal guidance specific to this issue, and your consultant's experience will help in this matter. Furthermore, keeping the conversation generic does not risk exposing the student's actions.

Option F: It may be wise to read the medical school's guidelines on plagiarism and they will likely provide some further guidance. Given that the student has unofficially submitted the document for review, it is more appropriate to act on an informal basis with the correct responses above. If the student had officially submitted the document, then it would be most appropriate to act according to the medical school's instructions.

Option G: By informing the medical school, you may prompt disciplinary action or a formal reprimand which may remain on the student's record. This is unnecessary at this stage, given that the student has not submitted the document formally. As he has only asked for a review, you should deal with this matter with the student personally. If the student later submits a plagiarised essay, it would then be appropriate to enact the guidelines.

Question 103

C, B, A, E, D

It is not practical to be able to avoid possessing sensitive patient data while working on the wards. Patient lists are integral to being able to work efficiently with all the key information about each of your patients and their jobs in your pocket. However, with this list comes the responsibility of safeguarding it from disclosure by handling it appropriately and securely. GMC guidance in 'Confidentiality' specifically states:

> You must make sure that any personal information about patients that you hold or control is effectively protected at all times against improper disclosure.

Unintentional disclosures may occur and in this scenario where a patient list has been lost, you must act sensibly to deal with the issues that will arise.

It is important to maintain your own integrity and probity, even at times where things have gone wrong and there exists the potential for legal or disciplinary consequences. Attempting to cover up a mistake may further compromise a patient's trust in the profession over and above the original adverse incident. It is important to escalate the matter quickly, once the list is confirmed as missing. A senior member of the team will then be able to offer advice on how to proceed, and the ensuing steps may involve notifying the patients who have been affected of the potential disclosure. While this risk to confidentiality always exists, you must take measures to minimise it by taking adequate precautions.

Option C: The first action should be to confirm that the patient list is in fact missing. It is thus best to ask the other staff present on the ward if they are aware of the location of the bag. This will avoid unnecessarily escalating the matter and causing panic.

Option B: A senior colleague should be notified at the earliest opportunity to enable the appropriate action to be undertaken. This may include informing other staff members to remain vigilant for the list, before notifying the patients affected about the potential breach. Given that preservation of patient confidentiality is more pressing than recovering your personal possessions, it is of greater importance to notify a senior in the first instance, before informing the police.

Option A: You should notify the police when a possession has been stolen. It is important to inform the police of the contents of the bag including the list. It is possible that the police may locate the bag and the list, averting any further damage. Before escalating the matter as far as the police, you should make a reasonable effort to confirm that your bag is indeed missing and that steps have been taken to limit the effect to patients.

Option E: Doing nothing is not a suitable response when confidentiality has potentially been breached. By acting early and taking measures to retrieve the list, there is scope to prevent harm to patients with the disclosure of personal information.

Option D: Misleading a senior colleague and keeping information from them actively prevents prompt effective management of the situation to limit the harm to patients. This is subordinate to Option E, in which your inaction does not deliberately foil attempts to control the incident. In addition, such deception is against the principles laid out by the GMC in 'Good Medical Practice' concerning the honesty and integrity associated with the profession.

Question 104

B, C, A, D, E

It is not uncommon to treat patients empirically while awaiting the results of further tests that may take longer to return. The concept ensures that the patient's disease or affliction does not worsen because you do not yet have all the information required to best direct treatment. However, just because the patient is receiving a treatment of sorts, does not permit you to neglect the results of the investigation. The concept remains that you are responsible for checking and acting upon tests that you have ordered unless an adequate handover to another suitable professional has occurred. This is of importance here, where you have learnt that the previous treatment you have prescribed is inadequate and the patient remains at risk of his urinary tract infection (UTI) worsening and potentially preventing him from having surgery. The best option is to hand over to the GP so that they can arrange an urgent appointment and manage the patient in the community. Given the failure in arranging this, the next most expedient option is to contact the patient directly.

Option B: Arranging for the patient to collect his new prescription from you at the hospital is the best option in the absence of handing over to the GP. This ensures that the patient's infection is treated as promptly as possible, although it is at the cost of your time which should be dedicated to your inpatients. It is worthy of note that the prescription that you provide must be for the hospital pharmacy only, and it would be good practice to inform a senior of your actions given that you should be prescribing under supervision as an FY1. FY1s are not permitted to use FP10 prescriptions without supervision, which are the green prescription pads used in the community. These would require completion under supervision or by an FY2 or above.

Option C: Asking the patient to attend A&E will also ensure rapid treatment for their UTI, and potentially avert cancellation of surgery. Casualty will have access to the urine culture results and will be able to deal with the issue appropriately. This option is subordinate to Option B, given that the patient will have to wait unnecessarily in A&E, for something which you can deal with quickly. Furthermore, it will still remain your responsibility to ensure that the patient did attend and receive the relevant antibiotics.

Option A: Calling the patient and asking him to see the GP means that the issue will be resolved within a reasonable amount of time. The GP will have to reassess the patient or else rely on the patient correctly informing them about the treatment in hospital. The GP's assessment will ensure that the patient has not come to harm and that further treatment remains their responsibility. As there is a greater delay in the time that the patient will have to wait for treatment, this response is ranked below the two above.

Option D: Sending a letter to the GP provides a prolonged unnecessary delay, within which period the patient may come to further harm, regardless of the quality of the handover. Although the GP will have better information than in Option A, the potential for the patient's condition to worsen without medical assessment, makes this response subordinate.

Option E: This scenario is not sufficiently severe to warrant cancellation of surgery. This is a simple matter in which the UTI requires proper treatment. Furthermore, this option neglects the patient's condition and the fact that it is resistant to the antibiotics he is taking, thus putting the patient at risk of his condition worsening without attention.

Question 105

A, B, G

Patients and their relatives may frequently question the management decisions made by your team. It is important that you understand the grounds for these, so that the correct justification for a seemingly obscure decision can be made. Being on the front line, you will have regular interactions with families and relatives who will raise difficult questions which you may be unable to answer. Such situations must be dealt with tactfully to avoid undermining the authority of a senior colleague and the stance of the team, while keeping the patient and their family fully informed. Contradicting previous management decisions without sanction, in the presence of the family, may compromise the faith they have in the care provided by your team.

This question highlights a scenario in which a senior decision has been made, which is not understood by both yourself and the relatives of the patient. The family are demanding the service concerned and as such it is important not to say anything that compromises the registrar to both the family and his superiors. While confronting your registrar about the issue may harm your working relationship with him and appear to question his authority, doing so from an educational perspective may allow you to learn about the salient factors in reaching this decision as well as provide sufficient information for you to relay to the patient and their family.

Option A: Communicating the decision the registrar has made to the family is important, as they should be informed of the latest developments. A conflict may arise due to this decision and specific concerns can then be addressed or relayed to the registrar, who may be in a position to provide further justification or review the initial decision which has been made.

Option B: The justification for the decision may be complex and it may be appropriate to escalate to a senior colleague to approach the patient and family, especially if you are uncomfortable with having this discussion yourself. Where conflict may ensue, the early involvement of a more senior colleague can prevent more serious consequences including a formal complaint being made or other medico-legal issues.

Option G: Approaching the registrar to gain greater insight into his decision will help you to learn the principles that can be applied to similar future cases, in addition to eliciting the necessary information to provide to the family.

Option C: Passing responsibility to another professional would be inappropriate. The ward sister does not possess any more information regarding the management decision and should not have a discussion which is better left to the medical team.

Option D: In instances where the registrar is unable to provide adequate justification for the decision which has been made, it would be appropriate to approach your consultant. While this may potentially harm your working relationship with the registrar, your top priority must remain the welfare of your patient. It is essential that you should approach your registrar in the first instance before escalating the issue to your consultant.

Option E: Exploring other management options may be appropriate, given that you are aiming to provide the best level of care possible in the instance that physiotherapy is not possible. Searching for an alternative does not address the issue at hand, however, and redirects the family's questions rather than dealing with them directly. As such this response is inferior to the ideal responses listed above.

Option F: Requesting physiotherapy input directly contravenes the registrar's decision, sending mixed messages to the family and undermines their belief in the medical team.

Option H: You are not in a position to recommend that the family seek private medical care. In addition, there may be reasons which are not clear to you as to why physiotherapy may be harmful to the patient.

Question 106

B, E, C, D, A

As a general rule, you should refrain from discussing patient information in public places even if the details are anonymised. The most innocent detail, which may not be an identifier such as a date of birth or name, may give away a patient's identity to someone who knows them. Items like patient lists should be safely guarded and, if possible, never removed from the hospital site, to prevent them from falling into the wrong hands. In this scenario, patient confidentiality is the central theme but when analysing the question, you must identify that patient care is also affected by some of the responses. When ranking the answers, it is clear that the best answers avoid discussing anything in public, followed by the responses that discuss details in an anonymised fashion, with the worst responses being those that involve discussing information freely. However, the manner in which the information is anonymously discussed should be scrutinised as some of them may compromise the handover you provide and consequently may affect the care of the patients that the registrar looks after over the weekend.

Option B: This is the best response in which you avoid discussing any details in public but address the matter in hand by providing an adequate handover. Phoning the registrar back when you are in a better environment will allow you to discuss the patients fully and provide a full handover with the benefit of your patient list.

Option E: It is best not to discuss anything at all on a busy train, given that you do not know who may be listening, hence the options below are superseded by this response. However, it does not address the issue of the registrar requiring an update on the sick patients and thus it ranks below Option B.

Option C: While not ideal, concealing the list and avoiding using names will help safeguard the patient's details when discussing them. Although confidentiality is compromised, you will be able to speak relatively freely and ensure that the information you impart is accurate and cannot be misconstrued thereby adversely affecting patient management. In contrast to the options below, this response favours a better handover, and consequently better care, over greater confidentiality and is therefore ranked higher.

Option D: Answering only yes and no without a list will make it more difficult for a third party to identify the patient that you are discussing. However, the trade-off is that you will be limited in the quality of your responses to questions and will be providing information from memory which may be inaccurate. This ultimately means that your information may be incorrect and misinterpreted, which may then adversely affect patient care. It is better to compromise on confidentiality than to risk harm to patients from an inadequate handover.

Option A: Discussing the patients without any attempt at anonymising them contravenes the guidance published by the GMC. It is not appropriate in any way to have this discussion on the train. Further to this, you are relying on your memory when providing your handover and this may affect the accuracy of the information. In summary, not only is confidentiality disregarded, but patient care is also compromised by an inadequate handover.

Question 107

D, B, C, A, E

It is difficult balancing training opportunities against working on the wards and completing jobs for patients, especially when these opportunities can be very infrequent. This is a dilemma faced by many SHOs with a keen interest in their speciality and sometimes it is easy for both them and you to lose sight of the fact that patients must remain the first priority.

You must identify in this scenario that the SHO's actions compromises the care that she provides for her patients and the cross-cover that you are providing will affect the quality of care for your patients, if not immediately, certainly in the long term as your cover is stretched. There are, however, further considerations as your actions must attempt to spare your relationship with the SHO, with whom you will continue to work, while aiming to reach a prompt resolution on the matter.

Option D: While it is important to maintain good working relationships, the issue must be dealt with directly. Discussing your concerns with your SHO should allow for an open dialogue on the matter and how it can be addressed.

Option B: Confronting your SHO is less appropriate as it is a more aggressive approach which may negatively impact on your working relationship. Such a stance may be detrimental when attempting to reach a compromise to this situation.

Option C: Escalating to the registrar is not ideal without attempting the options above, as it would bypass the SHO and constitute inappropriate escalation. Attempting to approach the registrar before speaking to the SHO will adversely affect your working relationship with her.

Option A: Requesting that other FY1s help you with your ward jobs potentially compromises the care that they provide for their own patients. It is not a long-term solution and fails to deal with the issue directly.

Option E: Refusing to perform the SHO's tasks is unprofessional and will harm patient care. It does not deal with the issue directly and will impact on your reputation with your team, as it fails to provide adequate reasoning for your actions. Regardless of the challenging nature of the situation, you should avoid any risk of compromising patient care, which should remain your first concern.

Question 108

C, F, H

Unnecessarily delaying a patient's discharge at their request is inappropriate and may be detrimental to a patient's well-being. This scenario is complicated by the offer of a bribe to prolong the stay in hospital.

Discharging elderly patients requires a multidisciplinary approach to ensure a safe discharge and the decision should not be undertaken by one individual. The discharge process itself should begin at admission with the involvement of all disciplines. Although your registrar has told you to discharge the patient, it remains your duty to ensure that the discharge is safe. The registrar may have read the entries from the other teams, but given the reluctance of the patient to go, it is important that you find out why.

Keeping the patient will mean blocking a bed and preventing another person from accessing the care they need. It also places the patient at risk of developing a hospital-acquired infection because of his stay. However, if the patient is not safe to be discharged, perhaps because there is no support at home, he is unable to mobilise or even does not have a home to go to, these risks must be accepted, otherwise the patient will return soon after discharge. Involvement of physiotherapists, occupational therapists and, if appropriate, social workers will prevent this from happening.

On the issue of the offer of money, it can be inferred from GMC guidance on probity that it is not acceptable in any form to accept this money as a bribe.

Option C: With the patient unwilling to go home, it is important to revisit the different aspects of his discharge. You should check from the notes that the other team members are happy and satisfied that the patient is safe to be discharged, before doing so. An inappropriate discharge may place the patient at risk of harm or may even precipitate a readmission shortly after he goes home.

Option F: Talking to the patient and exploring his concerns may go some way to reassuring the patient and enabling him to accept discharge. Alternatively, it may uncover a reason not to discharge the patient. It could be that the patient's normal support network is not in place, and in such a case it would be appropriate to hold discharge.

Option H: Discussing the case with other team members may highlight reasons not to discharge the patient, potentially averting an unsafe discharge. On the other hand, it may reassure you that discharge is indicated and there is no reason to keep the patient in. Your colleagues may be able to shed light on the reluctance of the patient to go home allowing you to address the issue.

Option A: While a physiotherapy assessment prior to discharge is important, there is no indication to specifically ask for one in this instance. Even if the patient is cleared by physiotherapy, this alone does not mean that the discharge is safe, given that the patient's home situation or functional abilities have not been clarified.

Option B: Deliberately holding up discharge in this way is underhand and dishonest. Inappropriately preventing discharge places the patient at risk of hospital-acquired infections and prevents the hospital bed from being allocated effectively. If the discharge is unsafe, it should be delayed in the proper manner.

Option D: This is inappropriate and against GMC guidance on probity.

Option E: Delaying the discharge on the patient's request alone without a proper reason is detrimental to the patient's well-being and may be contributing to institutionalisation.

Option G: There is no reason to ask for the patient to be reassessed at this point, given that no change in condition has been stated in the question.

The different teams will continue to work with patients once they receive a referral until they deem the patient to be back to baseline. If previous assessments deemed the patient suitable for discharge, there is no suggestion that there has been a change. Furthermore, it is not appropriate to tell a patient to donate his money to charity, as he may still perceive that he is paying for a service.

Question 109

D, E, A, C, B

Taking care of a dying patient can be very testing as it not only involves attending to the patient, but also liaising with the family, who may be conflicted among themselves at this difficult time. It is essential that the patient remains the centre of focus and his wishes fulfilled where possible, as opposed to his family's preferences. When a patient is identified to be dying, his wishes should be sensitively checked. Where this is not possible, the family should be asked if the patient expressed any preference. Regardless of whether or not the patient wanted to die at home, palliative care input is usually very useful and indispensable in facilitating a safe rapid discharge home. Although it is important to ascertain that a good support network exists at home, the palliative care team are the experts in such discharges and will promptly inform you as to whether such arrangements are feasible.

Option D: With the patient as your first priority, it is essential to check whether the patient had any preferences as to where he wants to die. Although the question states that the family wish for him to die at home, it is important to check with the patient that this is true where possible. If it is not practical to speak to the patient directly, then you should clarify with the family that the patient has either expressed or indicated that he would like to die at home.

Option E: Early involvement of the palliative care team will expedite the fulfilment of the patient's requests and help to optimise his care, whether or not he wishes to die in the hospital. Their input is invaluable and ranges from organising discharges to advising on appropriate medication.

Option A: Although a palliative care team will revisit this with the patient's family, it is important to know whether the family can manage at home with the additional care that can be provided. If the answer is no, then a discharge home may not be feasible.

Option C: Escalating to a senior is not required in this case. The end of life care or discharge should be co-ordinated between yourself, the nursing staff and the palliative care team. Senior advice should be sought when a complication or conflict arises, rather than as part of standard practice in this scenario.

Option B: It is not the case that large doses of morphine are an obstacle to a discharge home. Medication can be discussed with palliative care who can offer advice and support on suitable substitutions for regular treatment where required. Most medications are stopped towards the end of life, except those that are needed for symptomatic relief.

Question 110

C, E, A, B, D

The events outlined in the scenario demonstrate a lack of professionalism and may constitute sexual harassment. Your colleague is in a precarious situation where her superior is creating a tough atmosphere in which she is probably conscious that her actions may disturb the professional relationship that she has with both the consultant and the rest of the team. This is a common problem in the workplace and many advisory organisations exist to provide guidance and support. Legal recourse is an option, however, attempting to tackle the problem as locally as possible is often the best approach, with escalation if necessary. It may be wise to put things into writing or else keep a diary of events, should documentary evidence be required at any point. Close liaison with an organisation like the Citizens Advice Bureau will help to direct further action.

Option C: This is the most direct action in which your colleague can bring her unease to the consultant's attention. This action may prompt the consultant to stop making advances. If there is no resolution, it would be ideal to contact a relevant external organisation for further advice.

Option E: Taking action on your colleague's behalf without her knowledge or permission is not advised, and may damage your relationship with her. However, speaking to your registrar for further advice is the least intrusive option, minimising your impact on the issue.

Option A: Approaching the consultant directly yourself may unnecessarily compromise your colleague's relationship with both the consultant and yourself. Although it may help to resolve the problem, this should not be done without your colleague's permission, and may be inappropriate given that you may not be aware of the entire situation.

Option B: Reporting the consultant to the GMC is not appropriate and should not be done by you given that you do not have first-hand experience of the events that have taken place. This is a step in escalation which should be explored after local escalation within the hospital. This option is subordinate to Option A because of the ramifications of such an escalation based on hearsay.

Option D: This is another inappropriate escalation which you personally should not be instigating. There may be severe consequences from this action which may unnecessarily affect the consultant's career and registration with the GMC, given that they will be informed of any charges levied against the consultant. Your actions will further cause discord among the healthcare team.

C, E, B, D, A

Asking a team from another speciality to review a patient, with a view to modifying management is a frequent occurrence. While the review will highlight management options and yield recommendations, your team remains responsible for the care of the patient. This promotes continuity of care and ensures the best treatment, where the referring team knows the patient and their medical history best.

It is not normally the FY1's decision whether or not to enact these recommendations. This decision is usually undertaken by senior members of the team who also assume a level of responsibility for their actions. In this case, where the registrar has made a decision to ignore the surgical recommendations, this decision must be respected unless overturned by the consultant. It is likely that your registrar has a better understanding of why the suggested management should not be followed. It would be best to approach the registrar and attempt to understand the reasons for his decisions. It is not appropriate to bypass the registrar without good reason and escalate the matter to the consultant, especially when the consultant can be made aware of the situation during a ward round where the registrar can defend his position.

Option C: Attempting to understand the registrar's decision may go some way to satisfying yourself that the correct decision has been taken. Sensitively approaching the registrar will prevent any breakdown in the relationship between yourself and your colleague.

Option E: Approaching the surgical team will help to understand the logic behind their suggested plan and perhaps allow you to consider it in the context of your patient. It may convince you that your registrar is correct or may provide further reason and evidence to escalate the matter. It is better to approach your own registrar first given that he has better knowledge of the patient than the surgical team, and may take offence at you contacting them directly and bypassing him.

Option B: Discussing the plan with your consultant may create tension between you and the registrar. There may not be a need to bypass the registrar and it may be more appropriate to await the ward round where the registrar will likely explain his decision.

Option D: Requesting a repeat review does not change anything and may be wasting the surgical team's time as well as straining the relationship with your registrar, who has already given you instructions. There is unlikely to be any benefit from the review as the recommendations will likely remain unchanged.

Option A: Following the surgical team's plan is inappropriate. They are not responsible for the patient's care and your own team's advice should be followed. Your registrar knows the patient best and may be ignoring the plan because it is detrimental to the patient. If you take the decision to treat according to the surgical plan against instruction, you will be responsible for the outcome. In addition, ignoring your registrar will have a negative impact on your relationship with the registrar.

Question 112

A, C, E

'Raising and acting on concerns about patient safety', published by the GMC, states:

> All doctors have a duty to act when they believe patients' safety is at risk, or that patients' care is being compromised.

With this in mind, it is clear that your FY1 colleague is persistently making mistakes. The question does not state the severity of the other errors, but given that patient care is being compromised, you are duty-bound to act.

With the patient as your first priority, and in accordance with 'Good Medical Practice', you should endeavour to correct the error promptly, if you are competent to do so, averting any harm to patients. Consequently, GMC guidance states that 'you should first raise your concern with your manager ... such as the consultant in charge of the team', before suggesting appropriate escalation to other seniors in the Trust. Although these actions will affect the working relationship you have built with your colleague, you must place patient safety first, however, it would be wise to attempt to minimise the damage.

Option A: Talking to your own consultant is in keeping with GMC guidance as opposed to Option B. This should be done after correcting the error and minimising the threat to the patient.
Option C: Informing your colleague of the mistake he has made will directly benefit the patient. Your colleague will be able to correct the error immediately. This is preferred to Option E, which may contribute to your colleague feeling undermined by your actions.
Option E: Correcting the error yourself prevents patient harm and should be among the first actions performed. The situation is better dealt with, however, by raising the error to your colleague's attention. This response is superior to those below, given that it directly addresses the issue.

Option B: Approaching your colleague's registrar would highlight the issue so that the relevant team is aware. It does not, however, agree with GMC guidance to the same extent as Option A where you are informing your own superior and not your colleague's. Furthermore, approaching your own consultant is less likely to affect the relationship between your colleague and his fellow team members.
Option D: Filling out an incident form is obligatory but should follow correcting the errors and highlighting the issues to your seniors.

Option F: Escalating the episode to the GMC is inappropriate given that the issue should be dealt with at a local level first.

Option G: Monitoring your colleague closely may help to prevent harm to patients in the short term, but it is not a long-term solution. Over a period of time, the additional responsibility may impact on the quality of treatment that you provide for your own patients.

Option H: Gaining further information from the other FY1s will not help in this situation, given that you already have valid grounds to raise concerns about your colleague's performance. Asking the other FY1s may adversely affect your colleague's relationship with them.

Question 113

C, D, B, A, E

Online social media, including social network sites and medical blogs, can obscure the distinction between the private and professional lives of doctors. Material that is intended only for friends or other health professionals may be viewed by an unintended audience, including patients, senior colleagues and employers. The advances in social media may allow for improved communication among clinicians regarding patient care and greater learning opportunities. However, disclosure of personal information without consent goes against GMC guidance and constitutes a confidentiality breach. In addition, despite efforts to ensure that patient details are anonymised, derogatory remarks may undermine the public trust in the profession.

Developing personal relationships with patients outside of the clinical setting can blur the doctor–patient boundary and may give rise to challenging situations. These include the acquisition of private information about patients that has not been disclosed in a clinical consultation, and patients requesting informal medical advice outside of work. Doctors should therefore decline friend requests sent by patients and avoid personal relationships with patients.

Option C: Discussing the scenario with the patient makes the reasons for declining the friend request clear to the patient. Entering online personal relationships with patients may potentially lead to transgressions in the doctor–patient relationship and impact on the trust the patient has placed in you as her doctor.

Option D: Rejecting the friend request would be appropriate. This response is ranked below the option above, since you do not explain to the patient your reasons for doing so. Making this clear to the patient will justify your actions and may deter her from making similar advances in the future with other clinicians.

Option B: You do not always have control over the photos which are uploaded, or the information that is posted about you online. Controlling your privacy settings goes some way towards limiting the information that you share with your friends and the online community. However, this is not infallible and some caution must be exercised given the privileges and responsibilities that doctors have. Accepting the patient's friend request may still allow her to view sensitive information about you or your colleagues.

Option A: This response is subordinate to that above, given that you accept the friend request without any review or change to your privacy settings. This may leave you and your colleagues exposed, as the patient may be able to see everything that is posted on your wall. This will impact on your professional relationship with the patient and may harm the trust she has in the profession.

Option E: Deactivating your account and no longer using it is a bit extreme. You are entitled to a personal life and to socialise with your friends. While it prevents the patient from gaining access to your profile through an accepted friend request, this response fails to deal with the issue directly and unnecessarily impacts on you.

Question 114

B, A, D, C, E

An FY1's duties on-call will vary between different hospitals, however, in every hospital a chain of escalation exists whereby the SHO should be called for assistance before disturbing the medical registrar. The fact that the SHO is not answering his bleep when you need him means that a level of support is absent and that patient care is compromised to an extent. However, in such an event, your own intuition should prompt you to call the medical registrar if the SHO is unavailable and you are in need of assistance.

You should endeavour to resolve the issue as promptly as you have identified it. Ideally, you should inform the SHO that he should attend the relevant office and repair or replace his bleep, given that there is no indication that he is wilfully ignoring calls. Should you then suspect that the SHO is intentionally avoiding answering his bleep, it may be necessary to escalate the matter and relay your suspicions to the medical registrar. This step should not be taken lightly as such accusations will affect the professional relationship and trust among the on-call team. As patient safety is potentially compromised by the non-attendance of the SHO, the urgency of fixing the bleep should be impressed upon the SHO.

Option B: In the absence of an option advising the SHO to arrange a replacement of his bleep, the best option is to inform the medical registrar that the SHO is not able to respond to calls. The registrar may then be able to address the issue with the SHO and will know to expect calls from you that should normally be fielded by the SHO.

Option A: It is reasonable to call the registrar if you cannot reach the SHO when you are in need of assistance or advice. It is better to inform the registrar of the situation before an episode where you need help arises.

Option D: Although it is not advisable to escalate as far as the consultant early on, of the remaining options it is the only one that actively deals with the issue at hand. Enacting this, however, will strain the relationship that you are building with the SHO, and may affect the team dynamic. Ideally, you should always consult the registrar before actively contacting the consultant on-call.

Option C: Completing an incident form should only be done after the immediate issue has been resolved. Furthermore, while an issue with the SHO's bleep, or his willingness to answer it, has been identified, an event constituting a near miss has not been described. In addition, if patient care was involved, there is no reason why you could not have contacted the medical registrar when the SHO did not respond.

Option E: Gossiping with the other FY1s is inappropriate. It does not help to resolve the problems at hand, and furthermore it affects the SHO's working conditions and relationship with your colleagues. There is no evidence that the SHO in question is lazy – it is still possible that the bleep itself may have been faulty.

Question 115

E, A, C, D, B

Different hospitals have different policies on fielding calls from local GPs for the purpose of advice. In most places, it is the case that the on-call registrar is responsible for taking such calls. As an FY1 you should refrain from taking referrals or offering specialist advice given the potential consequences of your decisions. Such advice should only really be imparted by specialist registrars or above.

When considering the responses to this question, you should aim primarily to direct the call through the proper channels, and secondarily to minimise the time the GP is spending on the phone, although this should not be at the cost of patient care.

Option E: Strictly speaking, the registrar on-call is responsible for dealing with external calls. As such, the first port of call for the GP should be the medical registrar on-call or the renal registrar on-call if the service is provided. If the medical registrar is not able to provide assistance, he or she will then further direct the caller.

Option A: Although not an ideal escalation, putting the GP in contact with the consultant would ensure that the correct advice is offered. Asking the GP to speak to the consultant in the absence of your registrar follows the right chain of escalation. This response is preferred to Option C, where you are you not escalating appropriately within your own team, rather you are shifting responsibility to another team. It is also better than giving uneducated advice yourself, or wasting the GP's and your SHO's time by asking the SHO to field this call.

Option C: The GP should not be seeking advice from anyone less than a specialist registrar. In the absence of anyone in your own team who can address the issue, it would be appropriate to ask the GP to contact an alternate renal registrar.

Option D: Involving your FY2 would put them in the same predicament as yourself. Your FY2 would most likely have to explain that they are not able to offer any advice, wasting both their time and the GP's time. Furthermore, this is a needless handover of responsibility.

Option B: Offering advice yourself is inappropriate. Your advice may not be correct given your limited experience and may prompt the GP to act erroneously on bad advice, risking the patient's health. This is subordinate to Option D where your FY2 is unlikely to offer clinical advice.

Question 116

C, D, E

All allegations of child abuse must be taken seriously. It is important that doctors do not appear dismissive of a young person's claims. The GMC publication '0–18 years: guidance for all doctors' states:

> Children and young people are individuals with rights that should be respected. This means listening to them and taking into account what they have to say about things that affect them.

Doctors have a duty of care to their patients, including young people, and must ensure that their health and well-being is safeguarded and protected.

Option C: The on-call paediatric registrar is in an appropriate position to further investigate the issue and involve the relevant authorities. This response should be preceded by a thorough history and examination to fully understand what the child has reported and assess the severity of the claims.
Option D: Accurate and detailed documentation is needed to carefully record the allegations that are being made. It is likely that other health professionals and authorities will be involved and will need to review the precise allegations, including previous episodes and examination findings.
Option E: Having a nurse present during the consultation may provide extra support to the child and allows for a witness to the claims the child is making. However, the situation must be judged carefully to ensure that the presence of additional members does not make the child feel uneasy or less inclined to disclose information.

Option A: It is important to maintain a supportive and empathetic atmosphere when speaking to a child about sensitive issues. Questions should not come across as confrontational, as this may prevent the child from opening up about what has happened. Allegations of abuse must be taken seriously and it is essential to elicit as much detail as possible about what the child has experienced.

Option B: The child has disclosed the information when you are alone with him, and it would be inappropriate to have the discussion with the parents and child together. You must also respect the patient's right to confidentiality, and the same principles apply here as they do when the patient is an adult. Without the trust that confidentiality brings, the child may be less inclined to reveal all the necessary information.

Option F: You must not imply or accuse the child of lying. Allegations of abuse should be followed up with a thorough investigation and you should believe a child that talks about abuse.

Option G: There are more appropriate actions that should be undertaken in the immediate term, which include safeguarding the child. It is your duty to escalate your concerns to your seniors, which will allow for an investigation to take place. Reviewing previous admissions may reveal past injuries or other forms of abuse. These investigations will, however, be performed by other authorities and it would not be necessary for you to do this yourself.

Option H: Actions which safeguard the child are the most appropriate responses in this scenario. Highlighting your concerns to your seniors will allow for the necessary investigations to take place. The GP may or may not have information that relates to the conduct of the parents towards the child, but this research will be conducted by other authorities.

Question 117

E, A, B, D, C

It is important to identify the risk to patient safety in this scenario, should she have the MRI scan. Where the scan is not possible, you must find the next most suitable alternative. This will require input preferably from the radiologist. Given that you are aware of the radiologist's impending annoyance at your interruption and the remote chance that it will affect your relationship with him, you should try your best to avoid speaking up, but this needs to be weighed against the interests of the patient. In this case, patient safety comes first and thus you should not hesitate to interrupt if there is no alternative.

Another consideration must be the delay you will cause to the patient and the quality of advice you receive by not volunteering the information at your disposal. By not mentioning the patient's metal work at the meeting and informing your consultant afterwards, the imaging advice will be limited. The consultant may not be able to suggest a suitable alternative to the MRI scan and thus you will have to approach the radiologist again, wasting valuable time. If the information that you volunteer about the metal work proves to be wrong, this is not an issue. The radiologist will likely offer an alternative form of imaging, however, when you learn that the patient does not have metal work, ordering an MRI will still be possible. Doublechecking the notes will again only waste time unnecessarily.

Option E: By discretely asking your registrar to disclose the information, you are ensuring that the patient is getting the best advice about imaging given her circumstance. By avoiding interrupting the radiologist yourself, and involving the registrar, you are securing the best outcome without compromising your relationship with the radiologist, or his advice.

Option A: While announcing that the patient has metal work may place you on a bad footing with the radiologist, it is better that this should happen than harm come to your patient because of an inappropriate MRI scan or inadequate choice of alternate imaging. Approaching the radiologist later with this information will cause delay to the scan and will not benefit from the combined expertise available at the meeting.

Option B: Informing your consultant of the metal implants after the meeting is not the best approach. The consultant will either tell you to further discuss the case with a radiologist or offer an alternate form of imaging, which is better done by the radiologist. This will cause a delay to the scan and may compromise the quality of advice you receive as the information did not come from the combined expertise available at the meeting.

Option D: Doublechecking the notes on information that you are sure about will only delay the scan and will mean that you cannot obtain the shared opinion of your consultant and the radiologist as available at the meeting. By raising your suspicions of metal work and stating uncertainty at the meeting, you will have received good advice including the first choice being an MRI and a suitable second choice if MRI is not possible. This would have reduced the delay.

Option C: Not mentioning your concerns and making assumptions of the radiologist is not appropriate when you know the patient best. If the radiologist has not expressed that he is aware of the metal work, you should take the occasion to inform him given the risk to the patient's safety if she truly does have metal work and undergoes an MRI scan.

Question 118

A, B, H

Honesty and integrity are important attributes in a doctor. This question centres upon your suspicions that your FY1 colleague and his seniors are being dishonest in their conduct. This specifically relates to GMC guidance in 'Good Medical Practice', which maintains that doctors must complete documents with probity. Against these accusations, you must weigh the impact of your actions and how they will affect your relationship and reputation among the other FY1s as well as your colleague and his seniors.

Immediately it should be noted that there is no evidence of any wrongdoing in the scenario. It only states that you have doubts about whether the assessments have truly been completed. Without evidence of any suspicious events, there is no reason to question the integrity of any of the people mentioned. There is furthermore no justification to do anything proactive, in the interests of patient safety, because a specific threat has not been mentioned. Given that this is the case, it is best to opt for responses that have the smallest effects on your colleague as there has not been any wrong-doing that you know of.

Option A: Speaking informally to your colleague will not have any ramifications. Whether or not he feels competent in the skill that he has completed does not actually affect his ability to perform them. Despite this, it may be an indication that perhaps he has not been properly assessed, however, this is by no means conclusive or gives reason to pursue the matter further.

Option B: There is currently no definite evidence of wrong-doing and thus no reason to take any action. Integrity should be assumed unless there is evidence to the contrary. Just because your colleague has completed assessments that you have not yet managed does not mean that there is anything amiss.

Option H: Asking your colleague's seniors to assess you will not have any effect on their practice or their relationship with you. Rather, it is an opportunity to complete your own assessments and additionally to ensure that they are assessing their FY1s before choosing to escalate your suspicions.

Option C: Informing the GMC about a number of doctors at this stage is very premature. You currently have no evidence of wrong-doing and, furthermore, escalation should initially be at a local level.

Option D: Speaking to your colleague's consultant is not wise. Given that your suspicions have no basis, there is no need to involve senior management.

Option E: While it is more appropriate to speak to your own consultant before your colleague's consultant, it is inadvisable to baselessly accuse your colleague of wrong-doing.

Option F: Speaking to your defence organisation is a good answer. It is better to seek their advice before taking any drastic action. Talking to them in confidence provides you with reliable and confidential guidance which will not affect your working relationship with any of your colleagues. It is, however, superseded by the more appropriate responses above given that there is no evidence of wrong-doing.

Option G: Confronting the doctors signing your colleague off is preferred to approaching a consultant or the GMC. Despite this, it does not remain a good response. There is no need to speak to them given that they have not done anything obviously wrong. This conversation will affect future working relations with these doctors.

E, A, C, B, D

Being included as an author on a publication can have many advantages in addition to bolstering a CV. However, being inappropriately named is unprofessional and against GMC guidance on integrity:

> *You must always be honest about your experience, qualifications and position, particularly when applying for posts.*

This means that you should not claim experience or credit for a publication to which you did not contribute. Furthermore, from the perspective of the genuine authors, the addition of a name has a diluting effect on their achievement and level of input into the piece of work.

The matter must be approached carefully and consideration paid to the feasibility of correcting the situation. Firstly, it would be pertinent to ascertain the contribution of these two authors, escalating as necessary, before deciding whether or not to include them. At this moment in time, you do not know whether or not these additional authors have in fact contributed. This may not always be possible, with the time constraints on submitting a piece. In this case it is better to include the suspect names than to omit them. The rationale for this is simply that after submitting the document you cannot add further names and may deprive a genuine contributor of recognition. However, if the names have been added inappropriately, although the amount of your apparent contribution is diminished, the additional authors can be instructed not to claim credit for this work and their names even conceivably removed, albeit with difficulty. Essentially, what this means is that the addition of names can be rectified, but the removal of names cannot.

Option E: The best option is to discuss the issue with the registrar who has included the names. He may be able to outline the contribution of these additional authors, which you may not be aware of. It is possible that the content provided by the registrar was in fact produced by these authors. Given your involvement is being co-ordinated by the registrar, he should be the first person you contact.

Option A: The next step is to escalate to your consultant, if you are unable to talk to the registrar. The consultant may not know the additional authors, given that the registrar may be leading the poster, but could perhaps act as an intermediary. For this reason, it is better to speak to the registrar responsible.

Option C: Including the names on the poster is almost the default position. It is safer to include them than to deprive them of their rightful credit. If the names are inappropriately added for any reason, the authors can be instructed not to take credit for the work in future.

Option B: It is not wise to contact the other two authors given that you are not acquainted with them. Your email may interrupt a correspondence or collaboration with your registrar and may unknowingly compromise another project. Given that they are your registrar's or consultant's contacts, you should approach these colleagues first, or alternatively include the authors' names on the poster instead of contacting them directly.

Option D: Removing the two names will create a situation that is very difficult to rectify. This will prevent the two authors from claiming or proving that they have contributed, if they truly have. It is easier to deal with being added to the poster incorrectly, than resolving a situation where genuine authors have been omitted.

Question 120

C, F, H

This scenario is familiar to all of us when we approach a patient about to conduct our first attempt at a skill. It is very tempting to avoid or redirect questions that compromise the opportunity for you to perform the procedure, but doing so may be perceived to be as dishonest as lying about your experiences. 'Good Medical Practice' highlights that 'you must always be honest about your experience, qualifications and position'. Redirecting frank questions about your experience may not be an overt lie, but is still deception and should be avoided even at the cost of the patient refusing to let you perform the lumbar puncture.

In reality, it is best to be honest with the patient and answer the question directly. You should attempt to build rapport and the patient's confidence in you, such that she permits you to perform the procedure. Most patients understand the need to learn first-hand and will consent in the knowledge that it is your first procedure. In this scenario, the patient has only asked a simple question and has not even indicated hesitance at this potentially being your first attempt.

Option C: It is important to answer the question asked. The patient needs to know that this is your first lumbar puncture so that she can make an informed decision about who performs the procedure. You should also reassure the patient that you are competent to perform the procedure under supervision should she let you.

Option F: It is important to get consent for you to perform the procedure. Emphasising that you will be supervised will reassure the patient.

Option H: You must tell the patient that she is the first person you are attempting the procedure on. Informing her that you have done so before on models may help to get her to agree to you performing the puncture.

Option A: This is a good response, however, it does not address the question as directly as Option H, and is not as reassuring given that supervision is not mentioned. Thus Option H is preferred.

Option B: This response involves lying to the patient about your experience and goes against GMC guidance.

Option D: While this option is reassuring to the patient, it does not address the question directly and does not ask for the patient's consent for you to perform the procedure as in the preferred options above. It states and suggests that you will be performing the lumbar puncture, rather than asking permission.

Option E: Asking for consent on behalf of the registrar to perform the procedure is not consent for you to do the lumbar puncture. This option is counter-intuitive as it removes the possibility of you having your first try.

Option G: This is inappropriate as it involves lying to the patient about her right to refuse to have the procedure done by you.

Question 121

C, D, B, A, E

Despite this 23-year-old man describing the same symptoms continually with no obvious pathological process, it is not wise to ignore his complaints. There may be occasions where educated patients may describe symptoms with a view to delaying discharge, however, you must take the patient's word as true and investigate without prejudice. In this case, even if the man's previous episodes of chest pain were fabricated, there is the possibility that this one may be genuine, and thus cannot afford to be missed. Thus, with the patient as your first concern, you must investigate fully. There may arise occasions where you are informed that a patient should not be investigated for a complaint. These decisions are normally made by seniors and should be documented in the notes. Such a decision, however, should not be taken by an FY1.

Option C: Given that the patient is in pain, the first step is to provide some relief. If the patient is unknown to you personally, a quick brief history of the pain is necessary to ensure correct and safe analgesia is chosen.

Option D: Before starting the investigations, a history and examination is necessary. This will focus your choice of investigation and may clarify on the cause of the pain, and whether it is truly the same as previous episodes. Despite the likelihood of the investigations returning as normal, you must always investigate in case there is a pathological process.

Option B: Calling the registrar and discussing the case may be useful. If it is felt that the chest pain is due to another cause, medical or otherwise, the registrar may decide that it is in the patient's interests not to investigate further. This step should be taken after dealing with the acute episode, as the patient's welfare must come first before further management.

Option A: It is inappropriate for you to take the decision not to investigate the patient. There is no guarantee that the investigations will return normal and a decision of this magnitude should be taken by a senior colleague.

Option E: While conservative management is more than that offered by Option A, this response also includes documenting that the patient is not for further investigation, which is a potentially dangerous act. You should not be writing something like this without senior sanction, given that it may prevent someone who does not know the patient from investigating a serious and genuine complaint. This action may bring the patient to serious harm.

Question 122

E, B, A, C, D

When obtaining consent or speaking to a patient with disabilities, you must make sure not to discriminate against them in any way because of their affliction. There is no suggestion in this scenario that the patient has diminished capacity in any way. While the patient cannot communicate normally, he is able to express a decision by the use of a language board. Delegating the responsibility for the patient's decision or making the decision yourself is thus absolutely inappropriate, given that 'No one else can make a decision on behalf of an adult who has capacity', as outlined by the GMC in 'Consent: patients and doctors making decisions together'.

In accordance with 'Good Medical Practice', it is important that you ensure, 'wherever practical, that arrangements are made to meet patients' language and communication needs'. Where possible you should afford the patient the time needed to communicate with them effectively. Sometimes this is not practical and the task itself should slot into your list of jobs according to priority, given that more urgent jobs concerning treatment of other patients may exist. If necessary, it is possible to delegate a task such as this to another professional '… provided you make sure that the person you delegate to is suitably trained and qualified'. Thus, while it is not ideal to hand this job over to a nurse because you may be unfairly passing on responsibility, it is a potential option and should be done if it is in the interests of the patient.

Option E: While taking the time to speak to the patient yourself is the best option, it is not an available response. The alternative is to ask a nurse to talk to the patient on your behalf. While this involves delegating your responsibility, experienced nurses are able to do this.

Option B: Asking the family to assist in communicating with the patient is possible. It is, however, better to ask a staff member before resorting to involving family due to the inconvenience caused and the possibility that the patient may not be able to communicate freely with a family member present. Before asking the next of kin to assist, the patient's permission should be sought.

Option A: While it is ideal to take the time to speak to the patient, this job should not be prioritised ahead of more important jobs. This task should be completed in order of importance and ranking it higher than necessary may compromise care to other patients.

Option C: Acting in the patient's best assumed interests is inappropriate given that the patient has capacity. There is no reason to question capacity in this scenario.

Option D: Asking the next of kin for advice is the worst response. Firstly, they are not able to make decisions for an adult who has capacity. Secondly, while Option C guarantees that you are acting in the patient's best interests, it cannot be discounted that the next of kin may act in their own interests. For this reason, Option C is preferred to this response.

Question 123

C, F, H

In the UK, the law states that a person, including a doctor, is not obliged to help another human who needs resuscitation or emergency assistance, unless that person has caused the problem in the first place. However, the GMC publication 'Good Medical Practice' states:

> In an emergency, wherever it arises, you must offer assistance, taking account of your own safety, your competence, and the availability of other options for care.

Therefore, if a doctor chooses not to get involved in helping someone who is in a position of need, they will not be sued, but could be reported to the GMC, due to breach of the code of practice.

The above scenario takes place outside the hospital grounds. When you do get involved in an emergency situation outside the clinical setting, you have a duty of care towards the patient and must therefore act in her best interests. If your intervention is detrimental to the patient, you may be legally liable, particularly if the patient is left in a worse state than if you had not intervened. If the alternative is death, then this is not an issue since any rational action you take aims to prevent this. In other instances, you should act with caution to ensure that the patient does not come to any additional harm as a result of your actions, compared to if you had not intervened at all. In the USA, Good Samaritan laws exist, which aim to protect those who tend to others who are in peril, although their jurisdiction varies across states.

Option C: As outlined by the GMC, you should offer assistance and attend to the casualty. Basic life support is unlikely to pose any risk and may be life-saving when performed correctly.

Option F: It would be appropriate to stay with the casualty to provide assistance as the situation evolves, and to allow an adequate handover to another medical professional when they arrive. This will allow a smooth transfer of care when the paramedics arrive and minimises delays in providing the patient with the relevant medical attention.

Option H: Before calling an ambulance, it would be appropriate to assess the patient. In the absence of this option, arranging for an ambulance to be in attendance would be the next step. This would allow further management by paramedics.

Option A: While this is within your legal rights, it contravenes GMC guidance and you should offer assistance where it is needed.

Option B: Starting CPR on the casualty may be detrimental, given that you have not properly assessed her in accordance with basic life support (BLS).

Option D: While it would be pertinent to assess the patient, leaving the scene does not allow for adequate handover to paramedics. Furthermore, while the patient is currently stable, she may deteriorate before further medical assistance arrives.

Option E: The friend may not be medically trained and as such, may not be well equipped to action your recommendations. Catching the bus would result in neglect of your duties to the casualty. While the question states that you have an early start, maintaining a healthy work/life balance is secondary to the welfare of patients.

Option G: Physically carrying the casualty to the emergency department may cause further harm, and may potentially result in injury to you, the casualty or her friend. If the patient requires further assistance, it would be safer and more expedient to call for an ambulance, while managing the patient in the interim.

Question 124

D, C, E, B, A

'Good Medical Practice' states:

> *You must be honest and objective when appraising or assessing the performance of colleagues, including … students. Patients will be put at risk if you describe as competent someone who has not reached or maintained a satisfactory standard of practice.*

With this in mind, it is clear that with the current state of the situation, it would be irresponsible to sign this student off. While there is a conception that third-year students have time to improve, by approving this student as competent, you would be condoning the student's behaviour and promoting it to continue into future years.

Option D: Exploring the reasons for the absence will help you to advise the student as to his next steps without actually signing him off. If he has been absent due to illness for instance, you could offer him the advice to speak to the consultant in order to reach a compromise, enabling him to progress past the current rotation.

Option C: This response allows you to assess the student if he is willing to demonstrate the commitment and enthusiasm to shadow you for a few days. This option allows you to endorse his competence, if he manages to prove it to you in the trial period. It will also reinforce that being absent will threaten his progression from a given placement.

Option E: Refusing to sign the student off should be the default stance, in accordance with GMC guidance. It is subordinate to the responses above, in which you do not sign the student off either but offer resolutions to the problem.

Option B: Escalating may be appropriate if you cannot reach a solution with the student. Escalating as far as the medical school may be premature and inappropriate given that the consultant of the firm should really be informed first. This response is preferred to Option A, given that you are not improperly endorsing the student's competence.

Option A: It would be inadvisable to sign this student off without evidence that he is indeed competent. This action opposes GMC guidance and is thus the least suitable answer.

Question 125

A, D, B, C, E

Refusing to take blood from a patient with a communicable disease is against GMC guidance in 'Good Medical Practice', which states:

> All patients are entitled to care and treatment to meet their clinical needs. You must not refuse to treat a patient because their medical condition may put you at risk. If a patient poses a risk to your health or safety, you should take all available steps to minimise the risk before providing treatment or making suitable alternative arrangements for treatment.

Assessing the situation, you should recognise that the bloods are urgent. Given that your colleague is refusing to do them, despite your efforts to change her mind, you must identify that there is a risk to patient welfare. For this reason, you should act to ensure that the patient is bled. Following this, it is appropriate to counsel and speak to your colleague about dealing with patients with communicable diseases, her responsibilities and steps that she can take to ensure her safety without compromising patient care.

Option A: Given that the blood test is urgent and your colleague is refusing to do it, you should bleed the patient yourself to ensure that patient care is not compromised. The patient is always your first priority.

Option D: Giving your colleague safety advice may help to convince her to bleed the patient herself on a future occasion. Of the available options below, this is the least likely to cause offence or strain the relationship between yourself and your colleague.

Option B: Informing your colleague that she is obliged to take blood from a patient with a communicable disease is appropriate and may avoid the issue needing escalation to a senior team member. This response, while necessary, may negatively affect the working environment between yourself and your colleague.

Option C: Accepting your colleague's decision is not advisable. You should inform your colleague that her actions are against GMC guidance, given that she may not be aware. Furthermore, the patient is placed at risk if your colleague continues to refuse to take blood on occasions when you are not available to rectify the situation.

Option E: Refusing to take the patient's blood is against GMC guidance. This response is subordinate to Option C since you are responsible for your own active refusal, while in Option C you passively accept your colleague's refusal, which ultimately remains her responsibility.

Question 126

D, B, C, A, E

In this scenario, you are treating a woman who is the victim of domestic violence who does not wish for the matter to be escalated. You must weigh up the risk to her safety with her right to confidentiality. As stated by the GMC:

> *Confidentiality is central to trust between doctors and patients. Without assurances about confidentiality, patients may be reluctant to seek medical attention or to give doctors the information they need in order to provide good care.*

You should aim to maintain confidentiality wherever possible, though disclosure may be necessary if this is in the best interests of the individual or society in general. This may be required if the patient was at risk of serious harm or death. Such action cannot be justified in this scenario, although it would be pertinent to advise the patient of the options that are available should she change her mind. While advice can be offered, it is important to remain non-judgemental and not try to influence the patient's decision.

Option D: While the patient has stated that she does not wish to press charges, you have a responsibility to ensure that she is aware of the available options. Rather than influencing her decision, this response allows the patient to decide what is best for her.

Option B: It is good practice to maintain detailed, accurate notes on your consultations. If the patient were to change her mind and the matter went to court, you may be required to give an account of her injuries and it is therefore important that these are documented. This response does not deal with the situation directly and is therefore subordinate to the option above.

Option C: The patient does not wish for any further action and there are insufficient grounds to break confidentiality. Going against the patient's wishes will compromise the trust she has placed in you and the healthcare profession and may impact on future consultations. Not doing anything is therefore more appropriate than the responses below.

Option A: Contacting the police would constitute a breach of confidentiality, and this action cannot be justified since it would be against the patient's wishes and there is no immediate risk of harm.

Option E: This is the least appropriate response since this action constitutes a breach of confidentiality and would put the patient at risk of further harm.

Question 127

D, C, E, A, B

While there is a need to ensure that the notes that you produce are clear and accurate, you must obtain the patient's consent in order to share personal information with other health professionals. Consent is usually implied, as patients are generally aware of the need to disclose this information in order to facilitate good medical care. The GMC states:

> You must respect the wishes of any patient who objects to particular information being shared with others providing care, except where this would put others at risk of death or serious harm.

The patient in this scenario has been newly diagnosed with HIV and it could be argued that the patient may put staff at the GP surgery at risk during exposure-prone procedures. This, however, is insufficient to break confidentiality and go against the patient's wishes and will adversely affect the faith the patient has in the healthcare team. In addition, there must be a discussion with the patient informing them that a disclosure is going to be made, before such an action is undertaken. While it may be in the patient's best interest to share this information with the GP in order to effectively manage and treat the patient's condition, this again does not provide sufficient grounds to break confidentiality.

Option D: It would be most appropriate to explain the reasons why it is in the patient's best interest to inform the GP of his diagnosis. This discussion would also allow for his concerns to be addressed and reassured that his consent will be sought if this information needed to be disclosed elsewhere. If the patient continues to refuse, you must respect his wishes, in accordance with GMC guidance.

Option C: This response is the next appropriate as you respect the patient's wish to avoid disclosing the information to the GP. There are insufficient grounds to break confidentiality and you must therefore respect the patient's wishes.

Option E: While it would be advisable to make clear the potential risk the patient poses as a reason for informing the GP, this is insufficient to go against the patient's wishes and break confidentiality. This response is preferable, however, to the options below, where the patient is not given a choice and confidentiality is breached.

Option A: Disregarding the patient's wishes and informing the GP, irrespective of what the patient wishes, would impact on the trust the patient has placed in you, in addition to breaching confidentiality.

Option B: This response involves being dishonest with the patient and breaking his right to confidentiality. This is the least appropriate option as your lack of integrity will also impact on the trust the patient has in you and the healthcare team.

Question 128

B, A, E, D, C

With the patient turning blue and demonstrating cyanosis in this scenario, it is clear that her health is at risk. Furthermore, the question indicates that the nurses also share your concerns. This is an occasion where, if necessary, you must compromise working relationships with colleagues, since the overriding concern is patient welfare with the gravity of the situation. A professional relationship that is damaged by your actions in this event can always be repaired, however, the same cannot be said for the patient's health.

The anaesthetist is the most qualified person in the scenario to deal with the issue, however, he continues to persist in attempting to intubate the patient, where the patient is showing signs of a worsening condition. It is important to ensure that the anaesthetist is aware of the patient's condition so that he is able to evaluate his options appropriately to choose what the next best course of action is. In this situation, you should act in synergy with your colleague to minimise any potential delays in management, and where you believe that the patient is at risk from ill-advised interventions, it is your duty to act in the patient's interests, even at the cost of your relationship with your colleague.

Option B: Given the possibility that the anaesthetist may not be aware that the patient is deteriorating, you should inform the anaesthetist of your observations so that he can make a decision about his next action with all the appropriate information. This option is unlikely to cause any discord between your colleague and yourself and may prompt him to move onto the most appropriate management.

Option A: As you are aware that the next step is a tracheostomy and that before it can be performed, the set needs preparation, it would be appropriate to get this ready. This action will save time and it also gives the anaesthetist a little while longer to obtain a secure airway with endotracheal intubation. By enacting Option E before readying the equipment, the anaesthetist would waste time preparing the set instead of attending to the patient.

Option E: Asking the anaesthetist to perform a tracheostomy will strain the relationship between you, but is necessary if you feel that it is in the patient's best interests. In order to preserve the relationship, it is better to update your colleague to impress upon him the patient's deterioration, but where this has failed, you must act promptly.

Option D: Offering to help by attempting intubation is not wise. If the consultant anaesthetist is unable to intubate, then it is very unlikely that you will be able to do so with your relative inexperience. This response is superior to Option C, given that an attempt to help is being made as opposed to watching the deterioration of a patient and refusing to act.

Option C: Doing nothing is not an option. You are aware that the patient is becoming hypoxic and should hasten to inform the anaesthetist, who may not be aware of the gravity of the situation as he is concentrating on securing the airway. By not acting, you are risking harm to the patient.

Question 129

D, E, G

When approached by a senior such as a consultant and asked to perform tasks, there is a feeling of compulsion to accept. When agreeing to complete additional tasks for another team, you must ensure that you do not compromise the care of the patients that you are responsible for, since you are accountable for their treatment and not the treatment of the patients belonging to another team. Additionally, if you find that you are unable to complete the jobs, it is vitally important that you hand back the jobs, such that they are not neglected and patient safety placed at risk.

In this scenario, you have effectively been caught in the middle of what may be a spat between two consultants. You have not strictly acted inappropriately by accepting the supplementary jobs, but you must endeavour to keep a good relationship within your own team. Even though your consultant is unhappy with your actions, given that you have done nothing wrong, there is no immediate need to hand back the jobs unless you are unable to complete them. It is, however, important to talk to both consultants with a view to preventing a situation like this from occurring again. Unnecessarily handing back jobs that you have accepted inappropriately shifts responsibility and may affect communication with the other team, whom you may have to approach at some point to provide cross-cover for you. In dealing with this scenario, you must firstly aim to preserve a good level of patient care, before safeguarding your relationship with both teams.

Option D: As you have already accepted responsibility for the jobs on that day, you should attempt to complete them unless doing so compromises the care to your own patients. Neglecting these jobs without informing the other team may cause harm to patients.

Option E: It is important to notify the visiting consultant that this arrangement is not a long-term solution, and should only be done if his team are exceptionally stretched. This will help clarify your role with the visiting consultant and will help maintain a good relationship with your consultant when you inform him of the particulars of the arrangement.

Option G: Privately speaking to the consultant will help to repair the damage to the professional relationship and inform him that your choice to help another team does not affect the care that his patients will receive.

Option A: Asking your consultant for advice on the jobs is not necessary. Your consultant can only respond in one of two ways – telling you to complete the jobs or return them. If you are told to return them, then you will negatively affect your relationship with the other team and hand over responsibility for jobs that you can complete.

Option B: Although your consultant has expressed that he is unhappy with you completing jobs for the other team, refusing to complete any future tasks will affect the relationship with the other team.

Option C: Calling the other team to hand back the jobs would be shifting responsibility unnecessarily, and may compromise patient care where the other team are very busy. Given that you have already accepted responsibility for the work, you should complete it unless there is good reason not to.

Option F: Completing the other team's tasks after completing your own is dangerous. Some of the other tasks may take priority over your own and should be completed with a view to arranging things in order of importance.

Option H: Similar to Option C, you should endeavour to complete the tasks that you have accepted instead of handing back responsibility. Handing back the jobs the next morning is inadvisable given that you do not know the progress of the other medical team, who may be free enough to tackle these jobs. It would thus be more appropriate to hand the non-urgent jobs back to the team as early as possible.

Question 130

C, D, E

The actions of colleagues may at times put you in challenging situations that threaten the integrity and professionalism that you must display as a doctor. The GMC states:

> You must make sure that your conduct at all times justifies your patients' trust in you and the public's trust in the profession.

If a colleague comes to work hungover, it is important that this does not compromise on the safety of patients, or the professional manner in which they must be dealt with. The welfare of patients must take priority, and if the state of a colleague threatens this then you must take action.

In this scenario, a colleague requires medication to provide symptomatic relief and continue with his job. Paracetamol is readily available in hospital, although taking from ward supplies affects supplies available for patients. However, rather than being unwell and more prone to making errors or leaving colleagues on the ward with inadequate cover at short notice, there may be an argument in favour of taking the medication from the ward, if this is managed appropriately and does not become a regular occurrence. In this scenario, there are other options available that do not involve removing hospital supplies. While it may be inadvisable to leave work at short notice, this action is preferred to exposing patients to a doctor who is unfit to work and prone to mistakes. If a colleague is unable to work due to his condition then action must be taken to ensure that patients are safeguarded.

Option C: Issuing the tablets from your own supply would provide your colleague with symptomatic relief. It also avoids taking medication off the ward that is meant for patients, which would be inappropriate.

Option D: Patient safety should remain your first concern. If this may be compromised due to your colleague's condition, it would be more appropriate for him to go home than to continue working. While this may leave the team understaffed, appropriate cover may be arranged or cross-cover offered by other colleagues. While this is not convenient, it would be more appropriate than compromising patient care because of an unfit colleague who is at risk of clinical errors.

Option E: This response makes clear to your colleague that his actions are unacceptable, and aims to avoid future recurrence. Treating patients and colleagues with professionalism is integral to the work of a doctor. Coming to work hungover increases the risk of errors and compromises patient care.

Option A: While it may be necessary to report your colleague to a senior, this action is superseded by those that involve dealing with your colleague directly. This should be attempted in the first instance, to avoid damaging your working relationship with him. It may then be necessary to escalate appropriately if your initial actions are futile.

Option B: Providing cover while your colleague recovers may impact on your own commitments and the care that you provide your own patients. It is not a sustainable solution and your colleague may depend on you to do the same in the future.

Option F: This involves taking medication from the ward supply that is intended for patients. By hiding your actions from the ward sister, this is performed in a dishonest manner and is therefore inappropriate. More suitable options exist, where you provide your colleague with medication from your own supply.

Option G: Giving IV fluids also removes supplies from the ward that are intended for patients. Your colleague can tolerate fluids orally and there are inadequate reasons to give them intravenously. Patients and other health professionals may see your colleague receiving IV fluids on the ward and this threatens to undermine the trust that they have in you and your colleague.

Option H: This response passes responsibility to another colleague when it could be handled more appropriately by you. The ward sister is also likely to be busy.

B, D, C, E, A

It is difficult to pluck up the courage and make a call that you know will either reflect badly upon you, or potentially result in your chastisement. While it is preferable to avoid such situations, cases may arise where this is unavoidable. The question states that the patient requires an urgent senior review. After stabilising the patient in the immediate setting, this means that you must obtain help from someone who is more senior with greater experience than yourself. Thus it is clear that you must choose between the undesirable options of calling a consultant, who is likely to shout at you, or the alternative of calling the registrar who has already informed you that he is busy and will probably be annoyed at you repeatedly calling him. Nonetheless, the patient must take priority and you must accept repercussions of making the call and the impact on your professional relationship.

When deciding between these options, the ideals of appropriate escalation should be borne in mind. While it is true that you have contacted the registrar and he has already refused to see the patient, the next step of escalation is to bypass him by calling the consultant and this will strain your professional relationship with two colleagues. Furthermore, should the registrar continue to refuse to see the patient, the option remains to call the consultant, whereas doing things in the reverse order is more difficult.

In summary, you must place the patient's care first before considering whether your actions constitute appropriate escalation, and the effects that your choices will have on your professional relationships with the consultant and the registrar.

Option B: Calling the registrar after completing his instructions is the most suitable escalation. Although the registrar has already refused to see the patient, he may change his mind since you have finished the precursory work and highlighted the urgency of the situation. This response is preferred to Option D, because bypassing the registrar may create a difficult working relationship between yourselves.

Option D: As a senior review is absolutely necessary, the next step after contacting the registrar is to involve the on-call consultant for advice. Of the options available, it is the only other response that has a view to obtaining a senior review, from an appropriate member of staff. Although the consultant may be angry at you, this is outweighed by the needs of the patient.

Option C: Asking the nurses for advice on whom to contact is unlikely to prove valuable. The nurses are less likely to know the specification of your work or the process of escalation better than you. Furthermore, the above two options constitute the two most appropriate means of obtaining a senior review, thus the nurses' advice will deviate from protocol and is subordinate.

Option E: Attempting to manage the patient yourself is risking the patient's safety. It can be inferred that managing the patient yourself is beyond your competency and should be avoided in place of a senior review. This is subordinate to Option C, in which the interaction with the nurses aims to provide the patient with care from a more senior person than yourself.

Option A: Waiting until 5pm is an unsuitable response. The question tells you that the review is required urgently and thus you should not delay unnecessarily as you may be risking the patient's life.

Question 132

B, D, C, E, A

In this scenario, a newly registered patient has come to the practice to request a repeat prescription. You have a limited knowledge of his past medical history and the drugs that he is taking. While it may be convenient to comply with the patient's request and arrange for the repeat prescription to be issued, this is not the safest option. It may have been some time since the patient was last reviewed and the drugs or their doses may need to be changed or stopped. This should be made clear to the patient and he should be reviewed by a senior. A senior colleague should be notified of the situation and they may be able to provide advice on the appropriate action. They may be able to see the patient to arrange for the repeat prescription to be issued. The GMC states:

> In providing care you must … prescribe drugs or treatment, including repeat prescriptions, only when you have adequate knowledge of the patient's health, and are satisfied that the drugs or treatment serve the patient's needs.

From the available responses the safest options would be to review the drugs that the patient is taking and obtain an accurate record from the previous GP. Requesting that the patient arranges an appointment at the earliest opportunity to be assessed is safer than to prescribe a course of drugs that may be taken inappropriately and lead to serious harm.

Option B: Reviewing the drugs that the patient is on may uncover any medication that may be harmful if omitted or taken in overdose. If the patient is on any medication that requires more urgent attention, this may govern how the situation is managed. The patient is new to the practice and their drugs and past medical history should be reviewed before a repeat prescription is issued. If the patient has a history of psychiatric illness, this may put them at increased risk of harm to himself.

Option D: Contacting the previous GP will give a reliable record of the medications that the patient is taking, their doses and indications. These details can be reviewed with the patient to ensure that they are still up to date since the last review by the previous GP. Obtaining a past medical history from the previous practice will also be of benefit, particularly if the patient has a known history of suicidal ideation or psychiatric illness.

Option C: The patient should be reviewed before their medication is reissued. Provided that there are no medications that may cause harm if omitted, this would be the most sensible course of action.

Option E: Arranging for a one-week supply to be issued may pose some risk to the patient, if the drugs are not indicated or taken inappropriately. If the patient were to have a history of psychiatric illness or suicidal ideation, they may take all the medication at once and cause serious harm.

Option A: Asking the patient to attend casualty fails to deal with the issue directly and passes responsibility to another health professional. This would result in inappropriate use of the services provided by an emergency department and will put them in the same position, where they are unaware of the patient's medications and past medical history. The attending clinician will face the same dilemma of advising the patient to arrange an appointment to see their GP or provide a short course until they can be reviewed.

Question 133

C, D, G

In the post-operative period, it is not unusual for patients to be slightly confused as a result of anaesthesia, especially if they are elderly. However, when informed that a patient is in distress, you should not assume to know the reason for the distress before going to see the patient. The scenario in this question is exceptionally vague and does not enlighten you as to the type of distress the patient is experiencing, although it is clear that she does require calming down since she is trying to pull out her cannula.

In these situations, familiar faces can be useful and you should not hesitate to ask for help in the interests of the patient. You must be careful and must judge the situation properly before asking help from family members, to prevent causing distress to them or going against what you believe would be the patient's wishes. In these cases, it is key to assess the patient and uncover a cause for the distress, before acting to resolve the issue at hand.

Option C: Talking to the nursing staff and the patient herself will help to reveal the cause for the patient's current condition. While post-operative confusion is the most likely cause, you must keep the patient's interests at heart and assess the patient for other obvious causes of confusion, including hypoxia, infection etc., clues for which will present in the patient's observations and clinical state. Other causes will need addressing and treating.

Option D: Informing a senior member of the team may not be necessary if the cause for the patient's state can be identified and treated as appropriate. This option is among the top responses, however, as it is preferred to the other options for the reasons stated below.

Option G: The patient is in need of calming down, given the description in the question of her attempting to remove her cannula. Asking the nursing staff to help is advisable as they may be familiar faces to the patient, and a pacified patient is easier to assess.

Option A: Removing the patient's cannula may help to calm the patient in the short term but is not a good idea. If you assess the patient to be confused for a different reason, hypovolemia for instance, you may require the cannula to treat the patient. Putting a new cannula into a confused patient at this point is a lot more difficult and may be more harmful to the patient should multiple attempts be required.

Option B: Calling the husband in before assessing the patient is not advisable. It may not be an ideal moment for the patient's partner to visit her and may cause serious distress to the family. If the patient does require treatment and a full assessment, this is made more difficult and uncomfortable for you by having the partner present.

Option E: Sedatives should only be used when the patient is at risk of harming herself or others around her. Pulling out her cannula is not significant harm warranting sedation, and thus sedation should not yet be given. Before embarking on this kind of action, you should endeavour to assess the patient as it may become impossible to uncover a cause after sedation with the patient unconscious, or further disorientated. It is preferable to calm the patient down using good communication.

Option F: There is currently no indication to give the patient analgesia. The patient may already be on appropriate medication and may not be in pain. Analgesia should be given only after an assessment. This is important since, if the patient is confused due to opiates, prescribing more opiates will only exacerbate the situation.

Option H: Although this is likely to be a transient phase, not doing anything is inappropriate as you may miss a more serious complication. Before deciding this is transient, you should assess the patient to confirm that this is the case.

Question 134

E, C, D, B, A

It is difficult to weigh up your options in this scenario without first prioritising the consequences of each action. A good three-way balance should be maintained between minimising the disturbance to others, harming your relationship with others, and resolving the disruption. It is clear that the best approach would be to tell the disruptive colleagues to cease talking directly, without involving or disturbing others. Where this is not possible, you should try to notify them of your request, while minimising the involvement of others, thus minimising the impact on your professional relationship. When reviewing your options, you should further attempt to preserve your working relationship with your colleagues, meaning that you must not unduly embarrass them by highlighting the problem to the speaker. Additionally, you should try not to disturb the speaker where possible. When considering these factors, doing nothing about the issue may in fact be better than other responses, which have greater consequences. The situation should therefore be carefully evaluated before any action is undertaken.

Option E: Asking the person behind you to pass on a message means that you have involved one further person in your actions. It minimises the disruption you cause to other members of the audience and will not have a significant impact on your professional relationship with the offenders, but has the drawback of involving another person and forcing a responsibility upon them.

Option C: Speaking directly to the FY1 colleagues will disturb more members of the audience and may cause greater embarrassment to you and your offending colleagues. Given that you are disturbing more than one person and the scope for a greater impact on your working relationship, it is better to ask one person to pass on a message as in Option E, than the actions suggested here.

Option D: Ignoring the issue means that you have not resolved the matter and may not have been able to follow the presentation. Approaching the FY1s afterwards will prevent this from occurring in future but you are likely to harm the professional relationship as much as in Option E, without the added benefits, which are also present in Option C.

Option B: This is not ideal, although you will have preserved your relationship with your FY1 colleagues. They may continue to act in this manner in future and it is better to slightly compromise your relationship to resolve this issue, hence this response is subordinate to the option above.

Option A: Highlighting the behaviour of the offending FY1s to the speaker is the least suitable approach. You will have disturbed the presenter and furthermore caused the most damage to the relationship between you and the other FY1s, as well as disrupting everyone in the room. Given the scale of potential fallout, it is better to ignore the issue and do nothing than to cause such great impact.

Question 135

C, D, F

Angry patients can be a challenge to manage appropriately, as there is concern about exacerbating these emotions by addressing issues directly. The most effective way of dealing with such situations is to explore the patient's grievances, while remaining calm, empathetic and professional. Careful listening contributes to defusing the patient's anger, and acknowledgment of their feelings helps to restore trust between doctor and patient. Interrupting the patient with personal opinions or arguments before they have been allowed to complete their story may further exacerbate the situation, resulting in a power struggle and further deterioration in their relationship with you and the healthcare team. Empathy is a helpful tool in addressing a patient's emotions. Anger may be an expression that is derived from a patient's struggle with a particular condition, towards the condition itself or due to the apprehension felt due to an impending operation or procedure. Exploring the patient's ideas and concerns may help to elucidate any issues that were previously unrecognised.

This scenario assesses your ability to problem solve and diffuse a difficult situation, where a patient is taking out his anger and frustration at you in a busy waiting room. He proceeds to cast judgement on your competency as a doctor. These instances may trigger a protective response, where you wish to remove yourself from the situation or reply back angrily to defend your reputation. However, remaining calm and professional is more likely to be successful and restore the patient's faith in you.

Option C: The patient has been waiting a long time to be seen and this is likely to worsen if you insist on waiting for the notes to become available before you call him in. While the consultation may take longer without access to recent clinic letters, you should be able to get the information you require from the history and examination. While performing these actions, any missing information can be added once the notes are found. The consultation is also an opportunity to address the patient's ideas and concerns; he may have other issues that have not yet been explored. In such instances, adequate information and reassurance can be provided to help restore the trust he has in you and the healthcare team.

Option D: While you are seeing the patient, asking the nurse to continue looking for the notes may allow you to have access to them before the end of the consultation.

Option F: When confronted with an angry patient who challenges your ability, it may trigger angry emotions within yourself or a desire to remove yourself from the situation. Acknowledging the patient's discontent and apologising for his negative experience will help to diffuse the situation.

Option A: There may be a temptation to contact a senior with every uncomfortable situation. However, you should have sufficient expertise to deal with this patient. Involving more people may be counterproductive and compromise the faith the patient has in the care that you provide. By addressing the patient's grievances directly and exploring his concerns, you may uncover other reasons for the patient's outburst. This may then strengthen the relationship you have with him.

Option B: Insisting that you have access to the patient's notes before seeing the patient may augment his negative feelings towards you. While it would be beneficial to have access to this information, you may be able to elicit the information you require from a thorough history and examination. Any additional information that is uncovered from the notes when they are found can be included afterwards.

Option E: This response implies that a confrontational stance is taken. Remaining defensive or arguing back will exacerbate the situation and not help the doctor–patient relationship. It would, however, be beneficial to explore the patient's grievances and address these.

Option G: The patient is due to have an operation next week and if he is not pre-assessed, the operation cannot proceed. A confrontational attitude will not help to diffuse the patient's anger and will adversely affect your relationship with him.

Option H: While it may be necessary to inform the patient that his behaviour is unacceptable, this is once again a confrontational stance that will not help to diffuse the situation. The patient may have underlying concerns and acknowledging his feelings will help him open up. This will allow for any problems to be addressed and builds a strong relationship between doctor and patient.

Question 136

C, D, B, A, E

As an FY1, you should refrain from undertaking tasks for which you are not competent, or with which you feel uncomfortable. Breaking bad news is a refined skill that takes many years to perfect and should not be attempted without training or coaching by someone senior. In this scenario, where you are not familiar with the case and are also uneasy, you should not break this news to the patient without supervision, at least under an experienced nurse. The patient may have questions, for which you should try to be prepared, and thus it would be sensible to consult the patient's notes and speak to other members of staff before approaching the patient, should you elect to do so.

When breaking the news, other basic practices should be observed, such as preventing disturbance by handing over your bleep if possible, giving information in small amounts, with preceding warning shots, and the appropriate use of silence to allow the patient to register the news. Breaking this news inappropriately may affect the patient's belief and trust in the profession, influencing their choices in further management and cause avoidable and unnecessary distress.

Option C: Given that you feel uncomfortable breaking the news, which should ideally be done by a senior, it is important that you highlight this to the consultant. The consultant may then offer advice or suggest that you refrain from informing the patient so that he is able to do so properly at a more convenient time later.

Option D: While it is better not to approach the patient with this information if you feel uncomfortable, it is not an available option. Of the three options where you do speak to the patient, it is best to consult the medical notes. The best overview of the clinical scenario can be found here and, furthermore, there is written evidence to support anything that you do say to the patient. Medical information present in the notes may not be known to the nursing staff, thus this is preferred to Option B, which should ideally be done in addition.

Option B: Approaching the nursing staff for information prior to speaking to the patient may provide valuable insight and details of the case. It is subordinate to the response above as the nurses information will be verbal information that cannot be backed up by documentation, and the nurses may not be fully apprised of the clinical details, which will affect the information that you tell the patient.

Option A: Informing the patient of the news without any precursory preparation is ill advised. It is best to know as much detail about the situation when speaking to the patient so that you are better able to answer questions and demonstrate familiarity with the patient to prevent the consultation feeling impersonal.

Option E: Telling the patient that the consultant will return in the afternoon, without any guarantee that he will, is the least suitable response. This may only feed the patient's anxiety, and should the consultant not return, make the task of breaking the bad news harder with greater scope to negatively affect the patient's relationship with the doctor. Providing false information in this way may damage the patient's trust in the profession, thus it is better to break the news yourself, than to potentially unintentionally mislead the patient.

Question 137

E, B, A, D, C

Doctors have a responsibility to ensure that their abilities are regularly honed and that they are familiar with the latest developments that affect their work. The GMC states:

> You must keep your knowledge and skills up to date throughout your working life ... You should regularly take part in educational activities that maintain and further develop your competence and performance.

While having a duty to your patients, weekly teaching takes place at fixed times and provided that your team are aware beforehand, they should be in a position to cover you when attending these sessions. Normally, bleeps are collected at the start of these sessions and you are alerted if there is an emergency that requires your immediate attention. In this scenario, you have arrived late and therefore forgotten to hand in your bleep. The dilemma you face is deciding on the appropriate action, as your bleep has just gone off. The GMC also states:

> In providing care you must ... be readily accessible when you are on duty.

It would therefore be inappropriate to switch off the bleep. You must therefore manage the situation to ensure that the necessary care and attention is given to your patients, while remaining in the teaching session if possible.

Option E: Answering the bleep allows for the call to be screened for an emergency. Explaining to the caller that you are in teaching, providing details of when you are likely to be free, and the contact details of your SHO allows for you to attend the remainder of the teaching session. As you have left the session temporarily, it would be sensible to hand in your bleep to the administration staff at this stage.

Option B: This response also involves leaving the teaching session temporarily. While handing responsibility to someone else, the administration staff can screen the bleeps that come in and advise anyone who tries to get in touch with you that they should either call back after teaching, or contact your SHO. This allows you to maintain a satisfactory attendance average, which is required for sign-off at the end of the year. This response is preferred to the option below where you do not re-attend the teaching session.

Option A: This response involves leaving the teaching session altogether to attend to the jobs that you have been asked to do. This action is unsustainable, as you must attend the teaching sessions that have been arranged for your own development in the training post, as well as for sign-off at the end of the year.

Option D: Ignoring the bleep is unprofessional. Your team or nurses on the ward may be trying to reach you in an emergency. This response is preferable to the option below as you continue to monitor the bleeps that come through to you.

Option C: This response goes against GMC guidance. Your team or other healthcare professionals may need to contact you in an emergency. You will have no record of the bleeps that you have received during the teaching session if it is switched off.

Question 138

D, B, E, C, A

Every effort should be made to ensure that clear, accurate and legible records are kept. Despite this, inaccurate past assessments of patients do not provide adequate justification to make amendments to previous entries in a patient's notes. Subsequent entries can be made, noting changes in a patient's condition in light of new results that have become available. In this scenario, your consultant has asked you to make a backdated alteration in the patient's notes. This is a challenging scenario, as refusal to do so may lead to reprisals by your senior. However, you are responsible for the decisions you make and therefore culpable if the issue is escalated.

Option D: Making a note of the conversation with the consultant may be necessary in case the issue is escalated and there are legal implications.

It would be advisable to contact your medical defence union for further guidance on the appropriate measures that should be taken.

Option B: Escalating the matter to a senior is the next most appropriate response. Having a private discussion with the consultant, explaining that you do not feel comfortable doing this should be undertaken prior to this. Given the available options, reporting the matter to the clinical director will allow for the matter to be investigated. They may also be in a position to advise you on further action.

Option E: It may be necessary to inform the GMC. Highlighting the issue to a senior will allow for the matter to be appropriately managed and for the GMC to be notified if necessary. Escalation should occur in a stepwise manner, and therefore this response is ranked after informing the clinical director.

Option C: It would be appropriate to inform the patient of any errors that are made, in accordance with GMC guidance. However, this option also involves informing the patient of the consultant's request to make changes in the patient's notes. This may have a damaging effect on the patient's trust in the care that your team provides and there may be legal implications if they were to escalate the issue. You should escalate the matter as necessary and allow for an investigation to take place, but allow your seniors to deal with legal aspects of the case.

Option A: Complying with the consultant's request to make changes to a previous entry would be dishonest and may threaten to bring the profession into disrepute. There may be serious consequences to doing this and it is therefore the least appropriate response.

Question 139

D, C, A, B, E

One of the most important skills as an FY1 is prioritising your jobs and making the most of your time. This scenario is pretty straightforward, although there is a challenge in ranking two potential emergencies. The learning point here is to complete tasks that concern patient care first, prioritising the cases that need the most urgent action. While the question states that you are unhappy to hand over tasks to the night team, you must not compromise care to minimise the jobs you hand over. Furthermore, it is better to be handing over trivial jobs that can wait rather than emergencies which you should have dealt with immediately. It is also important to safeguard a good work/life balance, which involves leaving on time and ensuring that you get adequate rest so that you can provide optimum care the next day – so you should hand over tasks that you could not complete as opposed to staying back later to complete them.

Option D: Hyperkalaemia is an emergency that requires immediate treatment, due to the risk of life-threatening arrhythmias. Since the blood tests were done earlier, you should check them as a matter of urgency and if necessary continue treatment, including cardio-protection with calcium gluconate.

Option C: Although this is an urgent case, the patient is already under suspicion of appendicitis, and the option states that the patient is receiving treatment. Once the diagnosis can be confirmed, the patient may be operated on. Although there are no hallmark features described to suggest a perforated appendix which would be an emergency, you should review the patient to exclude this, given that he is again complaining of pain. In addition, you should prescribe more effective analgesia, and seek a senior surgical opinion if necessary. With no immediate suggestion of an emergency, you should attend to the hyperkalaemia first.

Option A: This is a routine falls assessment for a patient. Given that the patient is clinically stable and appears to have fallen out of bed, the assessment is not urgent although it should be completed as soon as possible. The fall may have been precipitated by infection, cardiac or neurological causes – all of which should be excluded by taking a history, examining the patient and ordering tests where appropriate.

Option B: Cannulating a patient who has a two-hour window for antibiotics takes lower priority than patients who may be ill and need intervention, thus it is ranked lower than the above responses.

Option E: Speaking to family is of the lowest priority because it is not directly associated with patient care. Furthermore, the information you will be able to provide is limited given your unfamiliarity with the case. The family may need to be advised to return when the patient's regular team are present, if they have specific questions regarding management.

Question 140

A, E, D, C, B

It is worth pursuing this issue, since being made to work more hours than your colleagues who are being paid the same salary can feel grossly unfair. Action must be taken sensitively, however, as the other FY1s may not be happy to undertake more shifts and this may manifest as hostility towards you, affecting your working relationship. It is thus better to defer the matter to others in positions of authority to resolve the matter, rather than acting yourself. There is always recourse to a union, such as the BMA, who would be able to offer support and advice. The least appropriate action would be to boycott your additional shifts without prior consultation which would risk patient care and safety.

Option A: Medical staffing are responsible for the rota and are the best people to approach. They can either explain their decision or take action to remedy it. Speaking to them in confidence means that you avoid the risk of alienating your FY1 colleagues.

Option E: Your consultant is unlikely to be responsible for the rota but is responsible for your placement. As with any problem, this issue should be escalated to them. They may offer advice or act on the matter, consulting the relevant people.

Option D: Asking your colleagues to act to make the rota fairer is a possible course of action. If, however, they refuse and are then made to cover your shifts by medical staffing, there is a possibility that they may resent you for your hand in the matter. For this reason, it is better to defer the matter to a third party to act independently and impartially, resulting in the higher ranking of the above responses.

Option C: Although the rota is compliant with the contract and technically you can be forced to work the hours, it is still worth pursuing the issue on the subject of principles and maintaining an equal work/life balance with the other FY1s. It is better to ask the other FY1s as a last resort if they are willing to balance the rota, even if they eventually refuse, than to do nothing at all.

Option B: Not turning up to your shifts without warning is unacceptable. Technically, the hospital is within its rights to ask you to cover the shifts as you signed a compliant contract. There is thus no excuse to compromise patient safety and care. Thus it is better to do nothing about the rota than to be absent.

Question 141

E, D, A, B, C

There will be many occasions where you will be asked to complete tasks and follow instructions, and you may feel a compulsion to do so without question. However, in these situations, you must always employ common sense and act in the patient's best interests. For instance, in this scenario your senior has asked you to obtain a review from the medical registrar. The purpose of this request is to obtain a more specialised opinion on the respiratory distress experienced by the patient. As such, consulting the respiratory registrar will not be objected to by your registrar, and may in fact be preferred. Furthermore, it would be pertinent to ensure that you have all the information you require to impart to the registrar, including examination findings and x-ray findings. This will increase your efficiency and shorten the time before treatment for your patient, as well as maximising the medical registrar's time.

Option E: When seeking a medical review, you will need to provide basic information to aid management and diagnoses. One of the first things you will need to mention are the current examination findings. As such, you should examine the patient and prepare your findings before making the call to the registrar.

Option D: Given that this is a case where there has been a change in the patient's respiratory status, it is highly likely that you will be asked to order a chest x-ray. Ordering it before speaking to the registrar will pre-empt their request and, if already performed, will foreshorten the time the registrar takes to review your patient. This may prevent them asking for you to call back after the x-ray is completed, and will shorten the time before review and subsequent treatment.

Option A: Given that the surgical registrar has specifically asked for a review and you are aware that the medical registrar is too busy to come in person, it is a good idea to approach a suitably equivalent registrar. This option will fulfil the surgical registrar's request, relieve pressure from the medical registrar and will ensure that your patient receives the best review. It is better than seeking the medical registrar's verbal advice as it means that the patient is physically reviewed, which is more important than the surgical registrar's suggestion that the medical registrar should be involved.

Option B: Obtaining a medical registrar's opinion instead of a review deviates more significantly from the surgical registrar's advice than Option A above, and is thus subordinate. Furthermore, it is better from the perspective of the patient to have a medical registrar come and physically review the patient, rather than just provide an opinion over the phone.

Option C: Starting the patient on antibiotics without indication or evidence is not appropriate. Prescribing a course of antibiotics without excluding a pulmonary embolism (PE) or pulmonary oedema may detract from further investigation and risks the patient's health.

Question 142

A, C, D, E, B

In this complex scenario, you are faced with a consultant whom you believe is being dishonest and whose actions are potentially compromising the patient's care. When answering this question, your first thought must be for the patient's safety and you should choose the responses with this in mind. There is the secondary issue of probity on behalf of the vascular consultant. Should the vascular consultant truly be deceiving your consultant, he is being dishonest and contravening GMC guidelines. However, you should defer action in this case to your consultant who is more senior and will have the same information as you to hand.

Option A: Before making any accusations, you should attempt to clarify the facts without incriminating anyone. In order to do this, you should first speak to the patient and ask without implicating the vascular consultant if she did in fact express an aversion to moving wards. If she admits this, then no further escalation would be required.

Option C: Expressing your concerns to your consultant allows him to take the appropriate further action. This may include clarifying facts for a second time. The purpose in doing this is essentially to secure the best care for your patient, which would be under the treatment of the vascular team. Your consultant's intervention is the best way to secure this result.

Option D: With the patient as your first priority, you should aim to provide the best care to the patient. While the above options attempt to place the patient under the vascular team's care, failing this, you should obtain advice from them on how best to manage the patient.

Option E: Not acting on your suspicions does not improve your patient's care, but neither does it impact upon it.

Option B: Speaking out of turn to the vascular consultant is ill advised. Dealing with the vascular consultant is best left to your own consultant and furthermore establishing whether or not he was dishonest is secondary to the patient's care. Creating a negative atmosphere with the vascular consultant could even affect the patient's care if the relationship breaks down to the extent that it becomes difficult to ask for advice on management.

Question 143

A, C, D, E, B

Striking a good relationship with the nursing staff can prove invaluable when working on the wards, both in a routine and on-call capacity. There will be many occasions where you will have disagreements with other members of staff, however, it is important to be proactive in repairing any damage done. In this scenario, there is no suggestion that you are responsible for any wrong-doing, rather you have seemingly been met with unprovoked hostility. Despite this, you should endeavour to be polite and avoid confrontation. Of the responses available to you, only two involve positive action. The remaining three must be ranked according to the least amount of damage done. The primary consideration here is to preserve the professional relationship you have with the nurse, although this is superseded by patient care in just one of the options.

Option A: Exploring why the sister is angry will provide an opening to strike a conversation with her. Uncovering the reasons for hostility will help to address them and prevent altercations like this in the future. Furthermore, a better atmosphere between you and the nursing staff will make for a better quality of patient care.

Option C: Telling the sister why you were late is a good response, although it does not attempt to resolve the current situation. It moves away from the sister's current verbal response, by providing an explanation, even though you are not accountable to her for your actions elsewhere.

Option D: Telling the sister to complain is not ideal. Although it is unlikely to be an issue if she does, taking this avenue of action will not help to promote a good working environment with the nursing staff. This response is only marginally better than the responses below, which are more confrontational and lead to situations which are harder to recover from.

Option E: Making threats is not appropriate. While the sister has acted improperly, inflaming the situation further by promising a complaint will make it significantly worse. Making a threat is more confrontational than Option D, and is thus ranked lower.

Option B: Insisting that you will not complete jobs for patients directly risks the quality of their care. The patient should remain your first priority, meaning that you cannot refuse to treat. Eventually, this means that you will have to stand down if the sister does not change her attitude, or compromise on patient care, which is clearly unacceptable. With this in mind, such severe action should not be taken.

Question 144

D, C, E, B, A

Maintaining a healthy work/life balance is important. Consistently working longer hours than you are scheduled to can have detrimental effects, including on your health and social life. However, patient safety must always take priority. When considering your actions, you must evaluate the impact that they may have on patient care. While you are on-site and your bleep is turned on, you have a responsibility to answer it. The caller may be seeking you for information that is only known to you. It is also possible that the doctor to whom you have handed over needs further instruction. Having answered the bleep, it is essential to adequately assess the call. In the interests of maintaining a good work/life balance, you should forward the call to the on-call team who is responsible for providing adequate patient care after the end of your shift, since you have already handed over to them. Your personal involvement may be required in cases where your non-attendance will compromise a patient's safety.

Option D: Answering the call to assess the situation is the best response. Given that you are on-site when the bleep has gone off, you are expected to answer it. Neglecting to do so may compromise a patient's care specifically if you are directly involved in the case. If the call is non-urgent, you can offer advice to contact the on-call team.

Option C: Although you must answer the bleep, it is not advisable to take down the job details to hand them over yourself. This response entails taking responsibility for the handover to the on-call team and you must not leave until it is done. This could potentially mean that you stay on-site for as long as it takes for a member of the on-call team to respond to you. This response is superior, however, to those below as it ensures that the job is handed over, helping to preserve a good work/life balance, but also that the job does not slip the net and get neglected or lost in handover.

Option E: Doing the job regardless of its nature is not conducive to a healthy work/life balance. As your shift has finished, you should request that the caller contacts the on-call team after you have assessed the job and ensured that it does not require your attention specifically.

Option B: Electing to only complete the task if it is not complex is not appropriate. Should the task be complex, you have not offered a solution to the caller. This may mean that the caller does not contact the on-call team, in expectation of your attendance. Should you then not attend, a patient's care may be compromised.

Option A: Not answering the bleep is the most inappropriate response. Given that you do not know the nature of the call and remain on-site, you should respond to the bleep to at least assess it and offer advice to call the on-call team if it is suitable. It is possible that the caller may be an on-call doctor, who is attempting to clarify the handover you provided. If this is the case, not answering the bleep may be detrimental to patient care.

Question 145

B, C, D, E, A

Cheating on medical examinations leads to an unfair advantage that can result in unsuitable students qualifying as doctors. Patient safety may be compromised if someone who has not reached the appropriate standards is deemed fit to practise. Cheating also lends itself to undue improvements in job prospects as students who score more highly than they otherwise would in examinations will be bolstering their academic ranking when applying for a foundation post.

In this scenario, you are made aware of two students who have cheated in their examinations. The students belong to your team, and you may therefore have a degree of loyalty towards them. However, the overriding concern should be the safety of patients. The GMC states:

> Patients will be put at risk if you describe as competent someone who has not reached or maintained a satisfactory standard of practice.

You therefore have a duty to escalate the issue appropriately to ensure that it is investigated.

Option B: This is a matter that must be taken seriously and investigated by the medical school. This will involve contacting those that are known to be involved to review how they came into contact with the exam paper. This should aim to prevent similar breaches in the future, and a repeat examination being set if necessary.

Option C: This response will allow the matter to be highlighted to the medical school and investigated. This may not be as effective, as there is limited knowledge on those involved and the scale of the problem. Maintaining the anonymity of the students is not essential, since they are not being treated as patients in this scenario. In addition, withholding names may be interpreted as protecting those that have cheated in the examination.

Option D: The examination was set by the medical school and they are best suited to deal with all matters relating to it, including suspected breaches. However, approaching the undergraduate education department at your hospital may still be helpful as they will be able to escalate the issue to the relevant people. This is a more convoluted pathway and may result in unnecessary delays, and therefore this response is subordinate to those responses that involve contacting the medical school directly.

Option E: Informing the students that their actions were unacceptable makes an attempt at addressing the issue and preventing recurrence. However, the examination has already taken place and action must be taken to rectify the injustice to the other students who have prepared and sat the exam with their honesty and integrity intact.

Option A: While advice from a senior may help to guide your actions, the SHO will be of limited benefit when dealing with this scenario. As the FY1 you are likely to have more involvement with the medical students and undergraduate teaching. Simply informing your SHO does not guarantee that any action will be taken.

Question 146

D, C, E, A, B

While the circumstances in this scenario are testing and not ideal, should such an event ever occur, you must remember that you are acting under the authority of the consultant and with his sanction. Despite this, you must concentrate on patient safety and thus aim to prevent any harm from coming to the patients, even if your actions are over-cautious. Adopting this attitude may involve annoying your seniors or colleagues with persistent bleeps or an inappropriate acceptance of patients, but it is better to embrace this consequence, than to unintentionally harm patients. A further point of note is that, as an FY1, your work is supposed to be conducted under supervision and you do not possess the authority to independently discharge patients. Normally on a ward, FY1s discharge patients on the instruction of someone senior as opposed to making the decision themselves. This formality must continue to be observed despite this promotion to a more senior role.

Option D: Bleeping the registrar after assessing the patients to ask his opinion will allow you to discharge patients under his authority, should he instruct you to do so. Although he will be difficult to reach and may not respond if busy, his input will prevent patients unnecessarily or inappropriately being accepted onto the surgical take, which may prevent them from being accepted under a more appropriate team, such as a medical, gynaecological, orthopaedic or urological team.

Option C: All the referrals will need assessing in order to determine whether any emergency action is required. Given that you are an FY1 on surgery and have limited experience, and that you should not be discharging patients, it is better to accept all referrals than risk them being discharged entirely because you have inappropriately cleared them from a surgical perspective.

Option E: Although the orthopaedic surgeons will have general surgical experience and are in a position to offer advice, you should consult your own team before attempting to contact another. This response is subordinate to Option C only as it would not be suitable to discharge patients on orthopaedic advice given that you do not know the competency of the doctors, and that they will not be responsible for your decision to discharge. Thus it is more appropriate to accept all the patients and let your registrar decide the plan than to ask the orthopaedic team for advice.

Option A: By refusing some of the referrals, you may be implying that there is no surgical issue. You should not be making this call given your limited experience and your actions may lead to A&E inappropriately discharging patients on your refusal.

Option B: Despite A&E doctors insisting that a patient should be discharged, you do not have the authority to make this decision and should hence refrain from doing so. This response is subordinate to Option A because it guarantees that a given patient will be discharged on your advice, whereas the above option leaves scope for an A&E doctor to re-refer to another team.

Question 147

A, E, D, C, B

Treating doctors can be daunting, given their pre-existing medical knowledge and ability. They should be conferred the same rights as all patients, and treated with the same level of care and respect for confidentiality. You must, however, assess the potential risk to patients as a result of their condition. If they do pose a risk, you may need to break confidentiality after informing them of the need to do so. It is inadvisable to ask doctors who are patients to manage their problem themselves or perform their own assessment to determine if or when they pose a danger to patients. The GMC publication 'Good Medical Practice' states that:

> ... if your judgement or performance could be affected by a condition or its treatment, you must consult a suitably qualified colleague. You must ask for and follow their advice about investigations, treatment and changes to your practice that they consider necessary. You must not rely on your own assessment of the risk you pose to patients.

Option A: Assessing the situation would help to determine whether the doctor is at any immediate risk to his patients. If this is not the case, it would be appropriate to offer advice on sources of support and to suggest that he takes some time off. This would allow him to take a break from work and reduce his current levels of stress.

Option E: A senior may be able to offer advice on how the situation should be managed. If there are any concerns regarding patient safety, the experience of a senior colleague may help to assess this and decide on further action. The situation must be dealt with carefully since mismanagement may risk endangering patients or compromise the doctor's career.

Option D: This response suggests that no current action is required or undertaken. The doctor has confided in you and may benefit from further support. With an alcohol problem, the patient may lack insight into the magnitude of the problem, and is not appropriately positioned to assess the severity or the risk to patients. He may return only after patient safety has been compromised. Therefore, you may be implicated in any incidents that he is involved in as you had knowledge of his problem and allowed him to continue to work with patients.

Option C: Informing the GMC would constitute an inappropriate escalation of the matter. The patient has approached you in confidence and this action would damage the relationship you have with him. This response breaches the patient's right to confidentiality and may compromise on the trust he has in the care that you provide.

Option B: Contacting his employer to help assess the severity of the problem would be the least appropriate response. This would breach confidentiality without any justification, and the issue could be more appropriately assessed by speaking to the patient directly. In addition to affecting the trust he has in you, it also risks compromising the doctor's career and standing in his place of work.

Question 148

C, D, F

Being flexible and open to compromise is vital to effective teamwork and success in your career as a doctor. When a colleague makes a reasonable request for time off work you should aim to accommodate this where possible. Patient safety should be considered and, provided that this is not compromised, your efforts to facilitate this will be appreciated by your colleagues. There tends to be a strong sense of camaraderie among doctors, particularly with demanding work schedules. With the difficulties of arranging annual leave around an on-call rota, it is likely that you will on occasion have similar requests to make. When arranging cover, the GMC states:

> You must be satisfied that, when you are off duty, suitable arrangements have been made for your patients' medical care. These arrangements should include effective hand-over procedures, involving clear communication with healthcare colleagues.

In this scenario, your SHO wishes to leave early to attend a personal engagement. This is not unreasonable, provided that it is cleared with your seniors, there is adequate cover for patients from equivalent or higher grade staff, such as a registrar, and that this generosity is not abused.

Option C: This action allows you to review each patient in turn to ensure all the tasks that were assigned on the morning ward round are completed, and allows for patients that require the most urgent attention to be highlighted. It may also uncover any outstanding jobs that must be completed before the end of the day.

Option D: As part of your professional courtesy to your colleague it would be appropriate to permit her to leave once this is cleared with a senior. An adequate handover must take place to ensure that patient care is not compromised.

Option F: Senior colleagues should be kept informed of developments on the ward. While you may not have any issue with your SHO leaving early, this must first be sanctioned by your seniors. Your registrar or consultant may need the SHO to help them with jobs that you cannot cover yourself as a junior member of the team. Furthermore, registrars may themselves be official cover for the SHO in her absence, should the need arise. It would therefore be appropriate to seek their approval first.

Option A: While all the regular jobs have been completed, new jobs or emergencies may arise. This does not provide sufficient justification to ask the SHO to remain in hospital, particularly if she has other commitments. You should have sufficient training to deal with many of the common scenarios that may arise. Your registrar could also be contacted for advice or if anything more serious were to occur.

Option B: The on-call doctor will not start their shift until after regular hours. Therefore bleeps that were directed to the on-call doctor may not be answered in the next three hours before their shift begins. It is thus better for you to hold the SHO's bleep and deal with the calls, escalating to the registrar as necessary.

Option E: Telling the SHO that she should remain in hospital to complete the shift would be unreasonable, considering that all the jobs are complete and an adequate handover can be provided. If the request was approved by a senior colleague, insisting that the SHO should stay may harm your working relationship with her and deter your colleagues from assisting you when you are in a similar position in the future.

Option G: While it would be reasonable to allow the SHO to leave early, this should first be sanctioned by a senior colleague. If any problems arise that are outside your clinical competency, your registrar remains on-site and should be contacted.

Option H: If all the jobs are completed and an adequate handover can be provided, telling your consultant that the SHO is leaving early and the reason for this is unnecessary and inappropriate. If needed, it would be more appropriate for the SHO to inform your consultant herself. This response may attract some degree of disciplinary action which would adversely affect your working relationship with the SHO.

Question 149

D, A, B, C, E

It is important to include as much relevant information as possible when making a referral to another doctor. In this situation where you have been berated for making an inappropriate referral, it is not clear whether the registrar feels that it is inappropriate in its entirety or whether you have omitted information that is now colouring the registrar's opinion. Nonetheless, your priorities should remain the same. Initially, you need to ensure that your patient receives the best and most optimal care which involves obtaining advice from the registrar. After securing your patient's interests, it is important to salvage the relationship with the renal registrar, with whom you may continue to work in future. Even if you or the registrar feels that the referral was unnecessary, it may be the case that the consultant surgeon is looking to exclude something that eludes your relatively limited experience, and thus the review should still be obtained.

Option D: Although it would be best to start with a cursory apology, you must keep the patient as your first priority and secure advice from the registrar. You will only obtain the best advice by fully updating the registrar with all the information at hand, thus this is the preferred response.

Option A: It is important to disclose all the information to the registrar before seeking guidance, hence this option is subordinate to the response above. However, given that patient care is more important than placating the registrar, this option ranks above the remaining responses that concentrate on preserving a healthy working relationship with the renal registrar.

Option B: Apologising to the renal registrar who is aggrieved by your referral will help to maintain a good relationship with her and will help the next time you require assistance. Apologising and explaining your actions will deal with the current episode and situation at hand, and will go some way to placating the registrar.

Option C: Understanding why the registrar feels that the referral is inappropriate will help to avoid the same situation occurring again. It will help to educate you on the circumstances and information you need to have before consulting the renal team. While this action is advisable, it does not address the current situation and is for future events, thus it is ranked below Option B.

Option E: Being confrontational towards the registrar will not help matters. Although there is no excuse for her berating you, you should not make matters worse and inflame the situation. This action neither helps the patient nor your relationship with the renal registrar.

Question 150

E, B, A, D, C

It is not uncommon to be asked to perform a favour as described in this scenario. When responding to such requests, it is prudent to remember GMC guidance on treating friends and family although this does not strictly apply here. The housekeeper here has asked you to perform a task that is outside of your capacity as an on-call doctor. When considering your course of action, it is best to employ an element of judgement. You are not being asked to do anything controversial or dangerous, rather you are being asked to perform a simple routine task for which you are competent. Given that you are not busy, there is no real reason to decline.

Being on a general ward, when bleeding the housekeeper, you will probably be using the ward's equipment. You should ensure that you do not cause stock levels of equipment to fall to levels that would endanger patient care in your actions, thus it is best to clear your actions with the ward sister. The only other consideration is your responsibility to check the results of the tests that you have ordered. This does not apply in this situation as the test was ordered by the GP, who is responsible for the test. Furthermore, if the phlebotomists had obtained the sample, the responsibility would not lie with them, rather it would defer again to the GP.

Option E: Informing the ward sister before obtaining the sample is ideal given that you will be using the ward's equipment. It is unlikely that the sister will refuse unless the ward's stock is seriously low. Not only does bleeding the housekeeper allow her to eat, it reduces the time she will spend off the ward waiting in the phlebotomy department.

Option B: Given the situation, there is no reason to refuse to fulfil the housekeeper's request. Although you are not obliged to help, you are not busy and no harm is likely to come from this action. When obtaining the necessary equipment, it is best to ask permission, thus this response is subordinate to the response above.

Option A: Gathering the equipment from the phlebotomy department will ensure that the job diminishes the stock in the relevant department only. This action will, however, cost you time and effort and may be unnecessary if plenty of stock exists on a ward. If the ward insists that the stock you use is replenished, it is possible to pay a visit to the phlebotomy department later in order to pick up replacements for the materials you used. Given that the ward and the phlebotomy department are part of the same hospital, this is unlikely to be an issue.

Option D: It is reasonable to cite your main concern to be your actual patients if refusing to bleed the housekeeper. There is no real reason to refuse, however, in this scenario, even though you are within your rights to do so.

Option C: Just because you obtained the blood sample, does not mean that you are responsible for checking and acting on the results. This responsibility lies with the person ordering the tests, in this case the GP. This is the least suitable option because the justification for your actions is based on incorrect assumptions.